GET SEX FAST

for men

by

Joe Sky

For Questions or Coaching,
email Joe Sky:

Sky@GetSexFast.Org

ISBN-13: 978-0615684734 (Joe Sky)
ISBN-10: 0615684734

Cover image of girl: © Hibrida/Shutterstock.com

—

INTRO

WHY IS GETTING SEX FAST
SO IMPORTANT ???

HOW I CAME TO WRITE THIS BOOK
& WHY I WROTE THIS BOOK

GET SEX FAST

—

Middle of the Date (do this)
Interrupt Her (before she shuts you out)
Initiative (it's up to you)
Physical Contact
(there's nothing more powerful than touch)
Being Creative
(part of catching a woman, is using your mind)
Seal the Deal (Have Sex)

Energy (it's all connected, use that connection)
Tension = Attraction
(coming together is more likely if there is intrigue)
In-Person (being together is the whole point)
The Moment (it all happens right now)
Break Apart (make her want you)
Letting it Go (move on)
You Never Know (when you least expect it)

INTRO

Ever been talking to a woman you were attracted to and sense that she liked you too and that there was something else beneath the surface going on and that something else was possible between you two? Did it ever seem that she was being really, really friendly? Just a little more friendly than normal and get the hunch that she was trying to tell you something? That maybe something else was possible, but you just didn't know how to go about exploring it and didn't want to make an ass of yourself or blow it? So you didn't push it any further? Well guess what, a lot is going on beneath the surface in male/female interactions all the time. We are sexual creatures and women are very sexual beings that give us hints all the time that most men are not even aware of. Women are much more adept at reading and expressing things with body language and hidden messages in their words and tone of voice than men are. If you learn to pick up on these signals and cues, a whole other world opens up to you that you always dreamed of but maybe never thought possible. Or you may have only thought it was possible for rock-stars or famous people. Women give off these signs all the time and want sex just as much as men do. It's just that they have to be more discreet about it because of how society judges them. Learn to read the lingo of getting sex fast and what to do and how to act on it to get as much sex as you ever dreamed of, making new sex friends and having flings with women that you may have thought were out of reach to you. Yes, a lot of women, just like men, are available for flings and sexual experiences even if they are in relationships because they crave variety just like you. Life is not meant to be so limited and black and white as you may think or have been told. In *Get Sex Fast*, I will show you how to read these signs that women are giving out all the time. I'll give you simple & direct routines of how to approach them, what to say and how to progress to get all the sex that you want, either the same day you meet them or on the 1st date. Not all women are looking for relationships. Women, just like men, want to have fun and experience new things with new people all the time; just the same as you enjoy eating a variety of different types of food on a regular basis or trying something out of the ordinary every now and then. You can meet women everywhere you go. You don't need to go to a bar or a club or to some online dating website... You can simply approach women that you find attractive at the grocery store, the gym, or anywhere you see them.

There is an energy that connects everything and those feelings and desires that you have are part of that energy. If you feel something, then that feeling, or energy, is connected to what you want and what you want, wants to be had by you. It's all designed by our creator to be complete. You are not just some odd person with strange wishes and desires who is separate from everything else. You are meant to have what you desire. If you have the guts to follow that thread of desire, then all you need are some simple, straightforward ways to communicate those desires to the object of your desire. You just have to be able to express it to her in the right way and that's what I am here to show you how to do.

These women are all around us, all the time, and they are hungry for new sexual experiences and just waiting for you to approach them. You see, it all starts within you. If you have the desire, then you have what it takes. God did not put a desire within you, without the ability to fulfill that desire. You simply have to trust the feelings that are within you and follow them. They *will* lead you to what you want. All you need are the inner qualities of belief, passion and perseverance and you will get anything that you want in this life including sex with all kinds of attractive women. I will give the right understandings, mind-set, simple routines and key phrases that will unlock all kinds of doorways to your wildest dreams. All you have to do is be willing to give it a try and stick with it. Ever hear the saying, "Ask and You Shall Receive?" or "Seek and You Shall Find?" Well, these sayings are true, all you have to do is have faith and believe in what you want and keep going until you get it. It is all up to you. No one else can determine what is possible for you, except you. You are in direct contact with the same force that gave you those desires and wants you to have them. That force will work for you if you simply trust it and follow it. You must believe it before you see it. So take charge of your life and lets get on the road to getting to *Getting Sex Fast!!!*

WHY IS GETTING SEX FAST
SO IMPORTANT ???

Whether you want a relationship, just sex, or anything in between, then getting sex is the key. The reason for this is because what grabs a woman and keeps her, is her feelings for you, or her emotional connection to you. Her vagina is directly connected to her heart and her emotions. If you give her good sex (orgasm...), and do it repeatedly, then she will become emotionally attached to you.

So, if you want a relationship with her, then having regular sex with her will keep her attached to you. All women want sex. If you don't have sex with her, then she will either, get frustrated and leave you, put you in the 'Sucker, you're gonna wait a while and MAYBE you'll eventually get some if you play your cards right' category or she will put you into the 'Just friends' category and you will not get any after that. So, this is why it is so important to strike right away or you will lose her, or it will become much more difficult to get sex later. Also, you will spend much more of your time, effort and resources chasing her around if you wait.

You, as a guy, know right away whether you want to have sex with a woman or not, right? If you do and you are confident, then you go for it right away, and she knows this. Women make the decision of whether they will have sex with you almost instantly, when they first meet you. They can size you up very fast. This is why you have to go for it right away and depending on her response, you can make an intelligent decision of whether it's worth continuing to pursue her or not.

If she doesn't go for it right away and she continues to see you, then she has put you into the relationship category and it may take some time before you will get any sex, depending on her relationship style, and she will probably be having sex with other guys in the meantime, that she calls, "Friends." Not to mention, you will be spending time, effort and resources pursuing her until, maybe, you get it.

If it is only sex that you want from her, then this will be a waste of your time, effort & resources… This is why you need to go for it right away and if she doesn't go for it, then you simply move on. It's a numbers game and there are plenty of women out there. In fact, if she sees that you know what you want and you move on if you don't get it, she will have more respect for you and become more attracted to you.

If you want a relationship, but you don't get sex right away -- the more time, effort and resources you spend trying to get sex, will just give her that much more leverage and then she will always expect these things from you. If you do get sex from her after that, it doesn't mean that you will necessarily be getting sex all the time. You may get it here and there, but then have to wait periods of time in between, where you will have to give her more of what she's now become accustomed to.

This is why you see so many men with no balls these days, who are just whipped around by their women, because they didn't have the balls to go for it right away and the women knew this and took advantage of it. And guess what, these women will never be satisfied by their men, because their men don't have the balls to stand up to them and their women are the type that will fool around behind their back because they don't really respect their man and can never be satisfied by a man that they don't respect.

If you come along and know what you want and have the confidence to go for it right away and get it, then you will have control in the relationship. If you don't want a relationship, then you at least you will get sex and have some fun. Women that will sleep with you, without a relationship, *move fast!* You have to move quickly to catch them; otherwise your opportunity will be lost for good. If they want to have some fun, it's going to happen fast with a man that knows what he wants and is confident about it. This is why *Getting Sex Fast* is so important, because either way, you will have the power to choose what you want. If not, you're just, "Lucky," if you get some. This is why you want to have some kind of a game plan and know when to draw the line on how long you will wait for it.

The interesting thing too, oddly enough, is that even if you just want sex and are not interested in a relationship with her, if you give her good sex, she will actually consider you for a relationship before other guys that have been pursuing her for a while and have spent a lot of their resources on her. Isn't that interesting? You're just going for a casual lay and you have more power than someone who has been chasing her for weeks, months or even years.

HOW I CAME TO WRITE THIS BOOK
& WHY I WROTE THIS BOOK

I was born to parents that were much older than typical parents. They were in their mid-forties when they had me. Their generation was way before that of most parents with children my age and their behavior much more old-fashioned, not to mention that our family was very dysfunctional. We were not very close emotionally and there was very little in the form of physical affection. We rarely touched each other, hugged or said, "I love you." My parents were not that romantic, flirty or playful at all. It was a very cold environment. My parents never talked to me about girls or sex or anything like that and my father was very harsh and critical of me. It caused me to go into a shell and become very critical of myself. So I went into this shell, especially starting around puberty, when all those hormones and things were kicking in and other boys were starting to get into girls.

I didn't have any guidance in that area at all and didn't feel much love. I felt that something was wrong with me and had only experienced being hurt emotionally for trying to get close to anyone. All those feelings of being interested or attracted to the opposite sex were suppressed and I felt very awkward, so I bottled up all those feelings and avoided it.

I never had a girlfriend or started dating like typical teens, or even in my twenties. It really wasn't until my 30's that my transformation started. Luckily, by the grace of God, I got into massage therapy. It wasn't for the obvious reason of hooking up with women. It was because I went through many years of severe depression and someone told me about a healer that unblocked people emotionally by working on their body. So, I went to try him out and the results were amazing! It really opened me up a lot and I decided to follow in his path and thought massage therapy would be a great way of helping others.

It turned out that getting into massage really helped me out in the long run with women, even though I never went into it with that intention. I was so far gone and out of it socially and emotionally, I didn't have a clue of what was about to unfold.

As they say, God works in mysterious ways and I believe that you always get what you need for your growth and your purpose here. Somehow, God has designed things this way. It's truly amazing the way everything is all connected. There is definitely an intelligent life-force that everything is connected to and part of, and that life-force works with us and gives us clues that are all around us everyday. If we pay attention to them we will continue to become more aware and grow.

Not having a clue about women, sexuality or any of that, I got into massage therapy for other reasons unsuspecting of what would come. I was pretty naïve for the longest time and didn't realize that a lot of the women I massaged were actually hitting on me.

Then slowly it became more apparent to me that something else was going on here and that a lot of these women actually wanted more than just a massage. In my latter days of doing massage, I came to realize that maybe 70 or 80% of the women that came to me, were flirting with me in one way or another; mostly with body language, telling me that they wanted more than a massage. Out of curiosity, I once asked a female client, what percentage of women in a relationship would actually fool around and she said about 80%. However, I realized that acting upon this in my professional situation could lead to other problems, so I had to find another, more appropriate way to explore my sexuality and the sexuality of women that I desired.

I realized that most women who came to me for massage, regardless of their life situation or relationship status, were actually open to having sex very quickly if put in the right situation. You see, society has made it ok for men to sleep around, but not for women. They get a very negative label for it. So, women, will go to all lengths to cover their tracks and protect their reputation; but put them in a private room with a stranger that is turning them on and more likely than not, they would act on it, because they too, enjoy and want pleasure.

Understanding this, I knew there had to be a more direct way to go about getting sex than the whole traditional, drawn-out dating process. Before this, since I had no guidance in my earlier years, as far as meeting women and dating...I just assumed all the typical old fashioned romantic bullshit scenarios had to ensue in order to get sex. I thought it had to be this long drawn-out process of courtship. I thought you had to meet someone, ask them out to dinner...and pursue a relationship, to get sex (going through that whole nice guy routine...).

I didn't realize that it could be quick and easy and that women wanted the same things as guys, just that they had to be more secretive about it. You have to learn the right terminology and process to **Get Sex Fast,** but once you know it, it's like walking through a fruit orchard, feeling each piece of fruit to see if it's ripe, then plucking it off the tree and eating it. It's very simple and doesn't take long.

When fruit is ripe and ready to eaten, it is ready! All you have to do is pick it and eat it... Women just like men, get horny all the time and want to have sex. They too, like variety and get bored of the same thing. They like to try new things and have new experiences... They are just waiting for new guys to come up to them and go for it. It's what validates them as being an attractive woman and spices up their lives.

I know as men, a lot of times, we may find it hard to approach women and we get nervous…but it is just like any other habit that you have to force yourself to do at first. Once you get going and get used to the process, it will become second nature and automatic. You will regularly start meeting all kinds of women and having all kinds of new and wonderful experiences that will make your life truly amazing and exciting to live!

I will first give you some attitudes, beliefs and understandings that you should have, that will greatly help you in the process. I will then give you the lines and simple things to say that are very direct and to the point, that make approaching women easy, not a bunch of canned silly stuff that a lot of these pick-up artists tell you to say… You don't have to dress like a clown to get their attention or go through long elaborate routines to get them. Again, the whole idea is that if they are ripe, then they are ready for the picking. All you have to do is walk up to them as your normal self, communicate in a simple direct way, ask the right questions, and respond the right way.

You see, I also wrote this book because I have not seen any other information out there that is so simple and direct. If I would have had this information when I was much younger, it would have saved me a lot of time, money and hassle. I could have gotten what I wanted much sooner and not wasted so many years of my life. I cannot believe that there is nothing else out there that shows you the absolute bottom line basics like this book does. Every man who is not successful with women should definitely know these basic building blocks before trying to digest more complicated techniques. In fact, with these simple and direct methods you won't need all that other stuff that other people are trying to teach. You can simply be yourself, approach women and get what you want because you understand how it works.

I will also show you how to follow-up, using text messages, phone calls or emails if they don't want it right then and there. The whole process is very simple. In fact, if you make it too complicated they will see that you are trying too hard and not really being yourself, and it will turn them off. If you are comfortable with yourself and they are ready, then all you have to do is be straightforward and use the right key-words and phrases that I will give you.

These key-words and phrases took me years and much trial and error and reflection, approaching thousands of women to figure out. Each time I would walk away from a woman or situation, I would ponder it and the clues that she had left and I knew there had to be a simpler, faster and more direct way to get what I wanted. These are things that women don't necessarily want you to know and will never tell you. They want you to figure it out for yourself; so I have done the figuring for you. A lot of it, is knowing, that this stuff works and being confident in the way that you deliver it. She will see that you are confident because you understand the process and she will open up to you because she wants the same thing.

You see, with my methods you won't feel like an idiot using them because they are very simple and direct. You don't have to come up with all kinds of stories and crap to tell them that is not really you. You simply go through the right process, ask the right questions, and respond the right way and if she is ready to go, then she is ready to go.

NOW LET'S *GET SEX FAST !!!*

GET SEX FAST

In my opinion, getting sex fast, is when you get sex with a woman on the first day that you meet her or on the day of your first date. This is my goal with this material. Sometimes it may take a little longer, but for our intents and purposes, our goal is the get it as soon as possible with the least expenditure of time, effort or money. The idea is that if she wants sex and is ready to go, then she is ready to go and we want to grab that opportunity and take advantage of it right now!

UNDERSTANDINGS & ATTITUDES
(to have)

Everyone Wants Sex
(it's a built-in desire)

Women want sex just as much as men do. It's just that society has given them a bad rap if they are too outward about it, so they have to be discreet and typically, they wait for men to approach them. They try not to make it so obvious that they want it, so you as a man, have to become like a detective and look for the signs that they want it and act upon them right away.

Women get horny just like guys do and when they want it, they want it. If you make them wait too long, then they will get pissed off and close the door on your opportunity. You have to PAY ATTENTION and be sharp and pick up on their signs and clues and act upon them immediately! If you hesitate you will lose the opportunity. Women pick up on hesitation instantly and it signals that something is not right and they will back out of the situation even if they had told you that they would do something earlier. So never hesitate!

Women Like Variety Too
(it's the spice of life)

Just as with anything, people will get tired of the same exact thing over and over and are always craving new things. That is the nature of the universe and who we are. It is our nature to constantly expand and grow. This means to continually be doing new things and things in new ways. Once someone has had the same sex partner for so long and has been doing things the same way, they will naturally want to try something different just for the fun and excitement of it.

Sometimes too, the other partner will get bored and slack off and maybe get too busy with work or other activities and no longer be fulfilling their partners' desires. Naturally if a woman is bored and not being fulfilled, or even if she is happy with her partner, it is still natural to want to try new things. Many women, who are in relationships, have sex with different men on occasion to fulfill their sexual hunger for variety.

It's also a biological fact, that for survival of the species, women crave variety and are always searching for dominant genes to reproduce with. It's built into their DNA. Most of being dominant is in your beliefs and attitude. Your beliefs are the deepest core of who you really are. Your attitude, body language and behavior, including Confidence, are a reflection of your deepest beliefs about yourself and Life; including whether or not you feel that you are worthy of having sex with a woman. Women pick up on this instantly, so you must believe fully in yourself and your ability to have her. Just having the balls to approach a woman that you find attractive will let her know that you are more dominant than 90% of guys, who don't have the guts.

You will be amazed at some of the opportunities that you will get just by simply approaching women on a regular basis!

It's a Numbers Game
(keep going)

Finding a woman to score with is a process. You are not necessarily going score with the first woman that you approach. It's simply a numbers game. You may approach 10 women and get 2 or 3 phone numbers and maybe only end up hooking up with 1 of those and you never would have guessed which one it would end up being. Sometimes, it's the one you thought was the least likely to come through. This is why you always, just keep approaching women all the time. The more you approach, the more chances you have.

It's a matter of approaching the right one at the right moment, and you never would have known that she was ready and wanting it until you approached her and found out. You never know, so just go.

Be Comfortable with Yourself
(Confidence)

Comfortableness equals confidence. You don't have to do a bunch of affirmations or anything trying to force yourself into believing that you are confident or somebody that you are not. You just have to accept yourself for who you are and go for what you want regardless. Yes, at first, it may be scary but you just have to push through that and keep going until you get past it. Eventually, it will become second nature and part of who you are without even thinking about it. It will just be something that you do and it will be an exciting gift every time you see a beautiful woman and approach her.

When you focus completely on the woman instead of yourself, you will get into her and into the situation and you will forget about yourself and just enjoy her presence. That is what makes the process so enjoyable, *her*.

Always Learning / Experimenting
(its Fun to see what happens!)

The whole process of meeting and seducing women
is FUN!!! And should always be fun! It's exciting to
be in a beautiful woman's presence and to interact
with her. Your focus should be on this and not on
how nervous you are or anything else. You need to
just focus on her and get into her. She will appreciate
this, as whoever she may or may not be with,
obviously, doesn't give her enough attention if she is
still craving it.

It is the attitude of Fun, Enjoyment and Pleasure that
you need to focus on. She will feel this if you are
focusing on it and she will enjoy this energy. This is
what will make her want to be around you. If she is
having Fun, then she will Enjoy being around you.

The whole thing is a learning process, just as with everything else. When you focus on the enjoyment of learning, it will inspire and motivate you to keep going. It is exciting to see yourself progress and get closer and closer to the goal you want: hot, beautiful pussy! The more you do it, the more exciting it will be to see your skills improve and to be getting what you want in all kinds of amazing situations that you never thought possible before, because you have the balls to keep going and are so fascinated with the process that it perpetuates itself and pretty soon it will become automatic. You will eventually become addicted to the process in a good way and it will not be a chore or difficult anymore. It will become an automatic response to seeing a beautiful woman. You will instantly want and have to go find out more about her by approaching and interacting with her. It will become so fun and enjoyable that you will find it difficult to stop, and each day will bring new excitement as you will be meeting more and more women all the time.

Like energies attract. The more that you go for it, the more your energy will continue to grow and you will naturally attract women because you are on a special frequency which they will detect and be drawn to.

Resistance / Testing (No, No, No, Yes)
(Don't listen to her!)

Women will always test you by resisting. They will not just simply let you have what you want easily without any challenge, but if you know what is going on and how to get past this then you can get what you want because you understand the process.

When a woman puts up some resistance, you do not just stop and walk away, you move around it. You dance with it and play with it until it becomes mesmerized by you and starts to dance with you. Women do like to dance, so if you dance with it, they will dance with you. Once they are enjoying the dance, they will give in because they do want it too. They just want it to be fun and enjoyable! You transform it with your sweet and smooth persistence. You do not approach it harshly or roughly.

Just because she may say no to something doesn't mean that you cannot ask something else or do something else or do it in a different way. So, that's exactly what you do. You keep going in a different way or at a different speed until you throw her resistance off and break through it and she melts and lets you have your way with her. If a woman is interested in you, she may say no several times, to different questions or actions but then as you gently persist, she will eventually give in.

One key is to notice her body language and how she is responding. If she is resisting or saying no, but she is still looking at you in a pleasant or open way, then most likely she is still interested and you should continue... For instance, if she is walking away from you but still looking back at you, then it may be that she would like you to follow her and continue trying, otherwise, she would just ignore you completely and not even be looking back at you. Pick up on these subtle body language cues and follow them more than what her verbal words are actually saying. Also, pay attention to her tone of voice. If it is a pleasant tone, then most likely she is ok with whatever you are doing.

Remember, Communication is approximately: 55% Body Language, 35% Tone of Voice and only 10% or less the actual Words that are spoken. So learn to pay attention to Body Language and Tone of Voice mostly. Whatever you do, if you are getting a warm, positive and friendly tone of voice and body language from her, then keep going ...

Women are infamous for playing games and trying to trick you out of what you want. Another way to look at what we men call, "Games," is to see it as a test, because that is exactly what women are doing. They are testing to see if you are stupid enough to listen to their words. If you do listen to their words, most times they will trick you out of getting sex from them. For instance, I swim laps for exercise and I had just walked into the pool area where I swim and I saw this attractive lady sitting on the edge of the pool getting ready to swim, I immediately walked right up to her, introduced myself, told her she was "Cute" and asked her if she wanted to join me for some "Coffee." She told me she didn't have time so I asked for her "Number," but she told me that she was in a relationship. So, I asked her if she wanted to be "Friends" and she perked up and got this big smile on her face and said, "Sure!" Then she immediately pointed to the water next to her and asked me if I was going to swim. If I was stupid and would have listened to her, I would have jumped in and started swimming. You see she was trying to trick me out of getting sex from her. If I would have got in and started swimming, I would have blown my chance of having sex with her. If a woman is not interested in a relationship and only wants sex right then, she may only give you that one chance and if you blow it, that may be it. Luckily, I didn't listen to her and instead of jumping in and swimming, I smiled and asked her if she wanted to "Come Over." She said ok, and we went back to my place and had sex.

Women Like To Be Chased
(start running)

It is a woman's job to resist and a man's job to open her. In order to do this, you must chase, follow, or pursue her and not give up until you get what you want. It's like all those sperms going for the egg and only one gets in. In order to be that one, you have to outdo the others and keep going. You must wear her out until she gives in and says, Yes! Just as in the *Resistance* section, a woman may say, "No" several times before she gives in and says, "Yes!" You have to have a sequence of several tries ready to execute until you get the, "Yes," you are waiting for. It's all part of the game, as she is not going to chase after you because that's your job as a man.

You have to become attuned to the signals she is giving off and not just listening to the words she is saying. It's a process that may take several attempts. Kind of like a wrestling match, where you're not necessarily going to pin your opponent on the first try. That's what makes it fun and enjoyable, is the challenge, the sport of it, and women definitely like to play. You have to be willing to play along with them. It's all part of the game. If you can enjoy the process, then you will be much more successful with women. Keep a good sense of humor about it. Smile, laugh and play along.

Women can tell if you have what it takes and they will even help you out at times if they see that you want them enough, because they too want the same thing. It's just that they don't want to be too easy and feel like a slut. So they have to play games to test you, to see if you want it enough. Also women have a disadvantage in the way that they can get pregnant. They have much more to risk. That's another reason they will test you with games. You have to have the balls to stick with it and show them that you have what it takes.

Women love to be chased. They want to feel wanted. If you give up too easily, they will feel that you are not that interested in them. For example, I have been swimming in the pool at my gym and talking to a woman in the next lane. I started a conversation and asked her out for coffee after, she said no and then I asked for her number and she said no. Later, as I was swimming, in the middle of the pool, she was leaving and she gave me this huge, playful smile and wave as she was walking away. I didn't realize it then but later it dawned on me that she was interested and wanted me to chase after her.

Another similar situation happened again. I was leaving the gym and this attractive woman was just getting there, as I was passing her, I asked if she wanted to join me for a drink and she kept walking past me but kept looking back at me with this pleasant look on her face. I was an idiot at the time, I left and later realized that I should have followed her and kept talking to her.

A lot of times when you are busy and in the middle of doing something, a woman will test to see how interested you are in her by seeing if she can get you to stop what you are doing and chase after her. This shows her how important she is to you. Women want to be number one. They will test to see if they are more important to you than whatever it is that you are doing at the moment. Society and men in general, typically value women for their beauty and attraction. In these terms, the most precious gift a woman can give you is sex. If she is going to give it to you, then she wants you to make *her* your #1 priority at that moment.

You also have to be able to read her and know when not to pursue her, or to let it go. In general, it's mostly about her body language, facial expressions and tone of voice. If she seems pleasant and is walking away from you, or just not giving in, then keep going and pursue her. If she starts to seem unpleasant or angry, then let her go. As time goes on you will get better and better at reading women. You will not succeed unless you are willing to fail miserably at first. Your results will get better and better as you go along and the progress will be very rewarding. There is nothing more satisfying or exciting than getting positive results with an attractive woman.

What Turns Her On
(your desire)

Unlike a guy, who can get turned on in a flash, like a light switch, just by looking at a woman, a woman, is more like a volume knob and has to be turned up gradually. A woman needs a reason to get turned on. She gets turned on by knowing that you are turned on by her. She wants to know what it is about herself that is turning you on and your passion for it. Women thrive on praise, and compliments work well. When you see her, pick something about her that you like and compliment her on it. It doesn't have to be a physical attribute either, it can be something about her personality, her brains or her taste in clothes. It can be anything, but try to be tactful about it. If you're daring and have a good sense of humor, then you can be more bold. Just experiment and see how she responds.

Attitude
(experiment & have fun!)

To become successful with women you have to have an open mind and continually experiment. Try new things and see how they respond. See what works and what doesn't. Most importantly, keep learning. Learning is fun and it should be fun to keep moving closer and closer to your goal.

You also want to take some time after each experience, at the end of the day or whenever and reflect on each situation that you had with each woman. Recall what you did and how she responded and ponder what may have worked better. As you ponder things and wonder about them -- new insights, intuitions and ideas will come to you. Continue to try these new ideas out and continually take note on what is working and what isn't and continue to refine your process. Ultimately, you are unique and you will eventually develop your own style that works for you.

You may have heard the phrase, "Seek & You Shall Find." If you keep trying and you don't give up, then you will eventually get what you want. Any goal that is worthwhile is never completely easy and without effort, but your life will be much better if you continue to go for what you want. In fact, if you want to be happy or satisfied in life, then you have no choice but to keep pursuing what it is that you want. If you just sit there and do nothing, even though you have desires and things that you want, then you will never be content. It is the continual *progress* towards that which you want, that gives satisfaction. It's not reaching your goal, though that is always great, it's the continual progress towards it. We always need something to do, and the pursuit of women and the process and mystery of seduction is definitely an intriguing and rewarding one.

It definitely can have its ups and downs, but if you keep moving and keep meeting new women, then you will continually have ups to look forward to and it will help you forget about the downs; not to mention, the accumulation of new female "friends."

I'm sure you've also heard the saying, "Ask & You Shall Receive." If you want the right answer, or the answers you are looking for, then you need to ask the right questions. Sometimes, all you need to do is ask the right question at the right time to a woman. After all, they are people too and sometimes want to be asked for that which is theirs.

The best way to be is to enjoy what you are doing and have FUN with it. Every heard the song by Cindy Lauper, "*Girls Just Wanna Have Fun?*" Well, it's true, they do like to have fun and fast sex is definitely meant to be fun! Having fun helps you to not be too attached to what you are doing. If you are too worried about the outcome, then it will not be very fun and it will inhibit your behavior and she will pick up on that. Women are very sharp and can usually read men much better than men can read women. If she senses that you care too much, or are too attached to getting it, then she may use that against you and you probably won't get sex anytime soon from her.

Physical Preparation
(neat & clean)

You must always do your best to be neat and clean at all times when approaching and interacting with women. As you can see, with most women, they are very particular about their own appearance. The least you can do is to be neat and clean when you are interacting with them. It is definitely a turn-off for them, if you are not. This includes: brushing and flossing your teeth and using mouth-wash regularly, keeping your hair neat and clean, and dressing decently.

I'm not saying you have to go out and get a new wardrobe or become someone else, just keep neat and clean and try to use good taste. It is important to remain true to yourself as well. She will pick up on it if you are trying to be someone that you're not and are not comfortable. If you are comfortable, then most likely she will be. If you feel awkward, you will probably make her feel awkward. Just try to be yourself, but with good taste.

The more in shape you can be the better. It shows that you care about yourself and women want to be with someone that cares about themselves. If you don't care about yourself, then she probably will think that you won't care much about her either. If you want to get a woman who has a nice body, then it doesn't hurt to be in shape yourself.

Do the best you can, otherwise don't worry about it.

APPROACHING

Anytime, Anywhere
(All the time)

You can approach women just about anytime and anywhere. In fact, I don't go to night clubs, bars, use dating websites or any of the typical places that most men think you have to meet a woman. I simply go about my life and do the things that I normally do, like going to the gym, grocery store, gas station, restaurant, coffee shop or wherever and if I see a woman that I find attractive, I approach her right then and there. In fact, to me, I think this is a much better way because you don't have to go out of your way, waste a bunch of time, dress how you normally wouldn't, spend extra money and do things that you normally wouldn't do and feel awkward.

I also think this is better because when you meet a woman who is out and about, say, doing her grocery shopping, for example. She is usually by herself, open and relaxed, her guard is down and she is not necessarily expecting to be hit on. You can just walk right up to her and do your thing. Whereas, at say, a nightclub…she will most likely be with her friends and maybe even a boyfriend, who at any time, may interrupt you, which so often happens. Actually weekdays, during the daytime can be especially good as everyone she knows is probably at school, working or busy and there is a good chance she is alone.

The gym can be an excellent place to meet women, which I highly recommend because you should workout regularly to keep in shape anyways. A man that is in shape is much more attractive to women. That being said, the gym is an excellent place because there are usually lots of women there and most of them are alone and not usually in a hurry to get anywhere because they are off work… You can simply walk up and talk to them. Also, a lot of gyms have hot tubs, saunas and swimming pools which are even better because women are just relaxing and you can relax with them and talk to them. Also, they are in their swimsuit and you are half naked which is way sexier and more suggestive... You can also go late in the evening to some gyms which is a great time because they are off work and may want to hook up and get laid before bed after a stressful day at work.

If you are at a fast food place, coffee shop or somewhere similar, these are excellent places if you see a woman there by herself and she is already sitting down, you can simply walk up to her and ask her if you can join her. Then just sit down and talk to her. If she is in line, you can ask her right there if she wants to sit together. This is perfect because it's an instant date. You didn't have to meet her somewhere, get her number, call her and figure out a time when you could both meet or any of that. You're meeting her and having your first date at the same time. Then since you already spent some time with her, she will already feel more comfortable with you and be much more likely to give you her phone number and see you again. She may even go home with you right then.

Just about anywhere that you see a beautiful woman or one you would like to bang, who is by herself, you can simply approach her right then and there, and skip having to go out to night clubs, bars or visiting internet dating sites and all that other stuff. This will give you so much more opportunities in your everyday life when you are least expecting it. This way you are in a pleasant state of surprise which she will sense and enjoy. Your energy will be much better this way. If you go somewhere expecting to meet a woman, you put a lot of pressure on yourself, which makes you more nervous and less likely to perform well. Also, if you meet them in your local area, then most likely, they live nearby too. That way, you don't have to deal with any inconvenient long distance relationships which will save you time and money.

In fact, women prefer to meet men in ordinary everyday situations, like when they are doing their grocery shopping, rather than at a night club where they don't trust the type of men they may meet there. They will see you in an ordinary, good light, rather than wondering if you're some kind of a player that goes to clubs all the time, drinks and hooks up with all kinds of women. They will see you as more of a normal, healthy guy.

Before You Approach
(scope it out)

Before you approach, you want to scan around to see if you notice anyone with her that may make the situation awkward, like a friend or boyfriend. If so, you may want to pick a different woman to approach. As I walk into a place or anywhere, I scan around and see if I spot anyone that I may want to approach and if it looks like she is with anyone.

There is also the *3 Second Rule:* once you see a woman you want to approach, you should approach her within 3 seconds. The reason for this is that the longer you wait and think about it, the more nervous and worked up with fear you will get and she will feel it. Whatever energy or feeling you have at the time you approach her will rub off on her and she will feel it. Don't wait, DO IT NOW!!!

Also, when you first see a beautiful woman, what state are you usually in? That's right-- Excited, Exhilarated, Passionate, Mesmerized, in a state of Wow or Wonder!!! You can use this to your advantage by approaching her Immediately! As I will clarify in a later section, energy is real and all around us; everything is made of it. The way that you feel, is the energy you are harnessing right now. Whatever state you are in, people around you can literally feel, especially women. They are much more in tune with it, in general, than men are. Since a woman can feel your energy, if you approach her immediately when you are in that wondrous state, she will feel this amazing energy and it will have a positive impact on her; even more-so than words. Use this to your advantage and save yourself the frustration of thinking about it too long and getting nervous. It will make your life much more fun, enjoyable and exciting!

Clues / Hints
(that she's ready)

There are certain things that will give you clues that women are, more likely, ready to be approached. I like to take an overall look at them at first and see what kind of image they are presenting. See how they are dressed: Is it revealing? Is it sexy? Do they have cleavage showing? Are they dressed excessively fancy or decorative? These may be signs that they are trying to attract more attention, which may mean that they are in the mood to be approached. I also like to see what colors they are wearing. Red is probably the biggest indicator of a woman feeling sexual. Also: Orange, Pink, and Yellow can signal that they would like to attract attention to themselves and be noticed, anything bright for obvious reasons because it attracts attention. I would say mostly in this order: Red, Pink, Orange, Yellow.

Pink, is a great one because it the color of their pussy, so there could be a little psychology behind it. In fact, I had a woman that had a crush on me who came over to do a presentation and share a business opportunity with me and she was wearing pink. I told her that I liked her pink shirt and she said, "Oh, you like pink?" She said it in a very flirty way and I knew exactly what she was talking about.

So, definitely colors and the way woman dress can be very revealing as to how they are feeling. Also, black can signify that they are not feeling the greatest at that moment. This too can be a sign that they may be open to something because they maybe in a relationship that is not going very well right then; which may be your opportunity to slip in there and give her what she needs.

Body language, obviously, is a big clue as to how she is feeling. They say it is 55% of actual communication. This is a subject that would definitely pay to study more. In general, if she looks open, there is more of a chance of connecting with her than if she looks closed off with her arms crossed, etc. Also, just by a general look at her facial expressions, you may be able to gather how she is feeling, if she looks friendly and in an open, cheerful mood, she probably is. Also, when you start talking to her, you will notice immediately how she is responding and you will know whether she sounds positive or negative. If she is sounding negative, then you probably don't even want to bother with her and just walk away. On the other hand, if she seems friendly and pleasant to interact with, is smiling, has pleasant facial expressions and a warm friendly tone of voice, then definitely go for it!!!

The overall vibe you are getting can tell you whether it's worth talking to her or not. If she doesn't seem interested then feel free to just walk away. Don't feel that you have to continue to try, it's a numbers game. This is the part where we start feeling the fruit to see if it is ripe. Some are, some aren't. If they are not, no big deal, just move on to the next one.

Also, if she makes eye contact with you and holds it for a few seconds or makes eye contact with you more than once, this is definitely good. If she does, then smile and see if she returns the smile. If she does, that's a definite sign that she is open to you approaching her. Also, if a woman is interested in you, she may put herself in your line of vision. She will want you to notice her. If you notice a woman in your vicinity more than once, then there is a good chance that she is trying to get your attention...

If they are interested, they will find any way possible to attract your attention. If she's with a friend and wants you to notice her, she may become kind of loud with her friend or they may start laughing just to show you that she is a fun person to be around. If your attention keeps being drawn to a particular woman and you find her attractive, then approach her.

These are all outward signs that she may want to be approached. Also, if you just have a strong inner feeling about someone and you find her very attractive, then approach her, even if you don't notice any outward signs that she wants to be approached. The more attracted you are to her, the more likely she will be attracted to you because she will sense your attraction and it will turn her on. She will literally feel this energy and enjoy it, whether she shows it or not.

Special Note
(use discretion)

Note: If you are in a store or somewhere inside and you just approached someone, you may want to walk to a different area before you approach someone else. You don't necessarily want everyone that just saw you picking up on a woman to see you hitting on other women. They may think that you are just there to hit on women and may not like it. Also, try to be careful not to do it too much in front of the employees. Once is ok, but if they see you hitting on multiple women while you are there, they may not like it and ask you to leave. Use a little discretion when approaching multiple women. As you go along, you will pick up on the vibes in different places. Trust your instincts and if it feels like that is enough for right then and there, then take off and move to a different spot.

Also, become good at acting aloof or kind of out of it, with a neutral or poker-face after you have talked to a woman and go back to what you were doing; or pretend that you are doing something else, like looking at things in the store... That way it doesn't look like you are just hitting on women. This is why I recommend just going about the things you would normally do and then when you see a woman that you are attracted to, you can stop what you are doing and approach her. This way, when you are done talking to her, you can go back to what you were doing and fit in.

Simple & Direct
(it shows more confidence)

It is best to be simple and direct in your approach. She already knows why you are approaching her, so it's best to just be direct. She will admire your courage and boldness and you will seem more confident which she will find attractive. No need to come up with elaborate stories, routines or any of that stuff.

You can simply approach her, introduce yourself, give her a compliment & ask her out to coffee or for her number... I will elaborate more on this in the *Routines* section and give you exact words you can say. Feel free to change your approach and words anytime and keep experimenting and trying new things. See what works for you. Ultimately, you want to create your own style that you are comfortable with, as we are all unique individuals.

It is also more fun to be bold and direct. At first, it may be kind of shocking to you, but it is definitely more exciting and you won't waste your time. You can simply approach and find out right away whether she is worth spending any more time on. If not, you can move on to the next one and save your energy.

Also, once you have a few experiences where you get far with a woman quickly, then you will get used to it and not want to go back to wasting time with long drawn out scenarios that waste your time, energy and money. That's only for suckers that don't have the balls to go directly for what they want. Woman will play along with whichever way you choose to do it, so save yourself the time, money and hassle. They will give you what you feel worthy of, and if you know what you want, then there is no need to waste time.

Tonality
(friendly & masculine)

The tonality of your voice is very important. As they say, it is approximately 35% of all communication. So you definitely want to use this to your advantage.

In general, you want a positive tone of voice: cheerful, playful, soft, warm, low… Again it depends on your exact style and what works for you, but overall, definitely a positive, warm tone. I tend to speak a little softer and quieter and found that sometimes that will melt women and get them to open up. It also depends on what kind of woman you are approaching and what kind of men she likes. I would say though, that since she is a woman, you should be a man and use a more masculine tone. Low and deep is usually good. Experiment and see what works for you.

Body Language
(open & masculine)

Just as with tonality, body language should be positive and open. Smiling is always a good thing that usually sets women more at ease and opens them up and they will usually smile back. Laughing can be good at times, but not too much. Overall, use open body postures. Keep your arms un-crossed, legs more open than closed, stand up straight, lean back, head high, make eye contact… Your glance, or gaze, at her should be soft and open, not harsh. Overall: warm, friendly, confident and open.

This is a good subject to do more studying on. The more you can read her body language and be aware of your own, in order to project a positive image, the better.

ROUTINES
(to *Get Sex Fast*, you must be Ready to Go!)

Key Phrases & Keywords
(to open the lock, you must use the right key)

"Coffee" – Coffee is a great standard keyword. After meeting a woman you can simply ask her to join you for some coffee. You don't actually have to drink coffee, but it is a pretty common term that lots of people use to refer to a casual, first-time meeting. It's simple and easy. You don't have to take her out to a fancy dinner, waste a bunch of money and time and set yourself up for an awkward experience if things aren't going well. There are Starbucks or other coffee places everywhere, that you can meet her. It's just an excuse to get things started with her.

Sometimes, when you ask a woman if she wants to have coffee with you, she may say no, or that she is too busy right then. This is when you ask for her "Number."

"Number" – "Can I get your number?" or "Let me get your number." Getting her number is key. You need to be able to get a hold of her. A lot of times when you meet a woman, she may be busy doing something and not have time right then to spend with you. So you have to have a way to get a hold of her and her phone number is usually the best way since women usually always have their cell phones with them. Sometimes she will offer an email address instead, tell you to stop by wherever she works or that she'll see you around, but her phone number is usually the best and most direct way to contact her. Sometimes, she may not want to give it out because she is in a relationship and she may not want her partner to know. In these cases sometimes, she will offer an email address or alternative way to contact her, but generally speaking, if a woman is really interested she will give you her number. Her cell phone number is the best to have since she will usually have it with her and you can then text-message her.

Sometimes when asking a woman for her number, she may say no or that she can't because she is in a relationship… This is when you ask her if she wants to be "Friends."

"Friends" – Friends is great term which makes it clear that you aren't looking for a relationship or anything serious, but opens up the possibility of having casual sex with her. You may talk to a woman and she may say that she is in a relationship or not looking for anything serious... Then you can ask her if she wants to be, "friends." She just may perk up with a big smile and say, "Ok!"
In which case, you ask her if she wants to "Come over."

"Come Over" or **"Wanna Come Over?"** -- Meaning of course, come over to my place, which of course, insinuates having sex. It is more appropriate and less awkward though, than asking if she wants to have sex with you. A lot of times, this is all that it will take to get her to come over and have sex with you when said at the right time.

Sometimes, after asking this question, she may say, "Why?" or "What are you thinking..." She may even say it in a deceptive tone which might make you think that she doesn't want it, but that is just her way of trying to trick you out of it or test to see if you have enough confidence to actually ask her if she wants to have sex.

In which case, you ask her, "Do you wanna have sex?" or "Do you wanna have some fun?"

"Sex" -- is of course what we all want and sometimes it can be as easy as just asking for it at the right time. Sometimes, a woman wants to know that you have the courage, or confidence to actually ask for what you want. After all, it is their most prized possession and the most valuable gift that she can give you. Women are taking a lot more risk than men when they have sex because they are the ones that can get pregnant and get stuck raising a child for the next 20 years. So, sometimes, they want you to have the balls to be able to ask for it. Sometimes, you will use the word, "Sex" to make a final clarification if she asks you what you mean when you ask her to come over or to have fun...

"Fun" – can also be used in place of, "Sex." You can also ask, "Do you wanna have some fun?" Instead of, "Do you wanna have sex?" Also, this is a more indirect way that is not as awkward and some women might appreciate this term instead, especially if they are in a relationship. They may feel bad answering, "Yes," if you ask them to have "Sex." In this case, having "Fun," may be more appropriate and when you say it with a flirty smile and tone of voice, she will know exactly what you are talking about. In any case, if she asks you what you mean, you can always smile and say, "Sex." If you want to be more indirect you can smile and say, "I give really good massages, you wanna come over?" Or even more indirect, "Wanna come over and play some cards?" If you go the more indirect way and they say no, then you can always break out the final question, "Wanna have sex?" It's up to you, just play with it and see what works for you.

"What do you do for fun?" – Women use this one a lot. It usually means that they want to have sex, but they want you to be the one to ask them. So, if you hear this one, then just smile and say, in a flirty tone, "Wanna have sex?"

"Are you happy?" --Women will also use this to see if you want to have sex. If they ask you this, then same thing as, "What do you do for fun?" You can ask them to come over or if they want to have sex… Or you can say, "You wanna make me happy?"

"Helping my friends out" – I've heard this one a few times. They may say that they like to, "Help their friends out…" It means that they like to help their friends Get Off (or cum)! If you hear this one, you will know that she is sexual. You can ask her if she can help you… If she asks you what for, you can say, "to relieve some stress…" or you can ask her if she wants to have some fun…

"Fling" or "1 Time Fling" – Some women who are in relationships may not want to give you their number, or be, "Friends," because they don't want their partner to find out and risk losing their relationship. However, they may be available for a one-time sexual experience or a "fling." If she doesn't want to give you her number or want to be friends, then you can always ask if she wants to have some fun, or is available for a fling.

"Have a Good Day!" (or **"Have a Good Night!"**) --
This is a good term to use, implying a double or extra meaning. Of course, in the standard sense, you are wishing them a good day, but in the extra sense, you are wishing that they have a Really, Really Good Day!!! Meaning of course, that you want to have sex with them. Ha Ha Ha! You want to use a little extra emphasis when you say this, again, a little flirty and playful.

*This is also a key phrase to listen for when she says it, especially when she says it playfully with a smile! In which case, immediately ask her if she wants to, "Come over…" Sometimes, she will give you a chance right then. If you miss it, it may be your last.

If for some reason you cannot follow up right then and ask her to come over, then either text her right away and ask her to come over or hit her up later that day or evening (including a late night booty call or text) and ask her; more on this in the Immediate Follow-Up Texting and Booty Calls/Texts sections.

"See You Soon!" – implies just what it suggests, except it has a more progressive edge to it. Sometimes when a woman texts you and says, "See you soon," she may just want to see you right then for the obvious reason. It's a little more suggestive than it may seem. If she says, "See you soon," then go ahead and ask her if she wants to come over right then.

Again, women are very tricky and manipulative and want to see how sharp you are and if you can catch these signs and hear what they are *really* saying. You have to be kind of a detective and always analyzing things, looking for their deeper meanings. Sometimes, it seems like they just want to play games and fuck with us guys, but they are testing us in one way or another. Just play along and see if you can understand what they are really saying... It's an adventure, so have fun with it!

"Next Time!" -- This is another tricky one that women use a lot. You may ask a woman out, either in person or texting and they may respond, by saying, "Next time." This means just what it says, but a lot of times, the next time may be right now! At first, I thought this had to mean another day or sometime later. I finally figured out that this was another tricky term that a lot of women use to see if you're going to catch it right then.

So, "Next time," can mean the next time you ask them which may be right after the 1st time, which is right now. However, you may want to phrase whatever you just said or did, slightly different. For instance, if you said, "Can I get your number?" And she said, "Next time," you could immediately say, "Ok, let me get your number."

I once met a lady at the gym, asked for her number and she said, "Next time." I said, "Ok, good meeting you," and then started to walk out because I was leaving. As I was walking out, I noticed she was walking right behind me and following me out. When I got outside, I turned around and said good bye to her again. Later, I realized that I should have asked her again or even better, I should have asked her if she wanted to "Come over." If she declined that, then I could have asked for her number again.

I definitely think that one of the best things to follow up with, when she says, "Next time," is to ask her if she wants to "Come over." That way you are not asking the exact same question in a row, but you are advancing it. A lot of times, women say "Next time," when they want you to ask them to come over. They want to let you know that they are interested and that you can skip that step and move ahead. You see, women have to be tricky like this because they can't be direct like a man, otherwise they would seem too forward and slutty and you probably wouldn't be as attracted to them then.

All of this is definitely a tricky game, but it is also a lot of fun and it is really cool to know that women do play these games and are willing to give it up if you play the game right. She may be in a relationship, but it's cool to know that a whole other level exists and if you play it right, then you can get things you never thought you could. So have fun and play!

"I'll See You Around" – A lot of women use this as yet another test to see if you are stupid enough to listen to them. Some may actually mean it, that they are not ready to hook up with you yet, so they put you off until another time when they run into you and are more ready or in the mood… Or maybe things are going well in their relationship, so they don't want anything else at the moment.

Sometimes, if you ask a woman out or for her number and she says that she will, "See you around," that can be another cue, just like, "Next time," and the question that you want to instantly ask her is, "You wanna come over?" Again, pay attention to her body language and tone of voice. If it is overwhelmingly positive, then go ahead and ask her if she wants to come over… You definitely won't get it if you don't try and if you don't ask!

"I'll Let You Know" – This one is similar to, "I'll see you around," or, "Next time." She may say this in response to some question you ask, like, "Wanna get some coffee?" or "Wanna come over?"… Of course, as with any of these phrases, she could be implying the typical meaning but it is also one of those tricky ones that can be used either way. For our purposes, we will go with the *tricky* meaning. Again, a lot of times, she is seeing if you're stupid enough to listen to her, when in actuality, she is letting you know right now. So, if you asked her to have some coffee and she said this, then ask her if she wants to come over. If you asked her to come over and she said this, then ask her if she wants to have some fun… Get it?

"Are You Ready To Go?" – If she does say yes to coming over or having sex, then you want to immediately ask her if she is ready to go and take off immediately! If you even hesitate a moment too long, she may completely change her mind. She wants a man that knows what he wants and is ready to take it immediately. If you don't value her that much, or are not that sure of yourself, then she will take it away just as quick. This is the fast track, if you want it quickly, without having to go through all the bullshit of ordinary dating, then you have to be ready for it and grab it immediately!

It's so quick and discreet that most men don't even know that this way exists. That's how clever and tricky women are. They are very good actors and good at covering their tracks. That's why they use all these double meanings with common terms. They don't want you to know, unless you are smart enough to figure it out; for 2 reasons: they want to breed with men who are smart and intelligent (which includes being quick-witted) and they don't want to be labeled a "slut," or mess up their relationship if they are in one, so everything has to be fast and discreet.

With all these keywords and phrases, or with any phrase or words that they may use, women are very tricky and want to see how sharp you are and if you are paying attention to see if you can figure things out. Trust your intuition and use your analytical and critical thinking skills. If you have a certain hunch or feeling about something that she just said, reflect on it and think about it. If you don't have time right then, then later when you are alone, laying in bed or wherever, think back over the situations that you've had with women, especially if they didn't go the way you wanted them to go and see if you can figure it out for the next time it happens. Ultimately, this is what you have to keep doing to improve your skills and abilities. This is how I figured these things out. In addition, of course, keep educating yourself with valuable materials, like this, that other people have already spent a great deal of time on. It will get you ahead that much quicker without having to go through all that headache yourself.

"Stress" -- Sometimes women will use this word as a sign that they want sexual release. If they say that they are really stressed and you are feeling bold, you can ask them if they want to have sex... If you don't want to be that bold, you can ask them if they want to come over or come over for a massage... If they say no to that, then you can then always ask them if they want to have sex.

"Where Do You Live?" -- This is a big time key phrase that a lot of women use to let you know that they want to come over and have sex. Keep your ears peeled for this one and once they ask it, give them a short description of where you live, making it sound close by and immediately respond with, "Do you wanna come over?" or "Let's go to my place!"

See, women don't want to seem like sluts, so they want to give you a clue or a hint and want you to bring it up, as if it were your idea… A lot of times, if a woman is attracted to you, she will ask you this during your first conversation, or sometimes she will ask it immediately on your first date. Say, for instance, you first date is getting coffee with her. She may ask you this just after you order the coffee and are waiting in line for it, or maybe even before you order. A lot of times, they are giving you a test to see how fast and alert you are. They are trying to catch you off-guard, since you might not be expecting it because you just got there. They will test you to see if you can catch it and respond correctly right away. Be very aware of this one! This is probably one of the biggest key phrases that they will say that indicates that they want to come over and have sex and a lot of times they will use this one right away.

"Are you going home now?" -- This is another clue that she wants you to ask her to come over… It is similar to, "Where do you live?" Treat it the same way and ask her to come over…

"What are you doing...?" -- Or anytime she asks you what you are going to do... It's another clear sign that she wants to get together, so go ahead and ask her over...

"Been busy?" -- or -- **"Have you been busy?"** If she asks you this, what she is really saying, is, have you been busy fucking... Women who are very sexual, get turned on thinking you have been busy with other women... It triggers the jealousy/attraction switch within them and makes them want you more. They want to be turned on, so they will ask you something that turns them on. All you have to do is smile and say yes or "mmm, hmmm," and ask them if they want to come over and have some fun!

"I like meeting new people" – This is pretty much the same as her saying that she likes fucking new people. It's another clue she is trying to give you. It's another open invitation for you to ask her to come over and have some fun... Similarly, she may ask you if you meet a lot of people... If so, just smile, say yes and ask her if she wants to come over...

"Why don't you give me your number?" -- A lot of times women will say this when you ask them for their phone number. This again, is another test. She is seeing if you are stupid enough to listen to her. If you give her your number instead of getting hers, she will not call you. Women do not call men. Very rarely do they ever, especially after you just met them. The woman expects you to pursue her. If she asks you this, you can say, "If I call your phone, then you will have my number in your phone." Or you can say, "Never-mind," casually and walk away and see if see changes her mind and says Ok. Be creative and think of different ways you can respond to these things. Women are always testing us to see if we are going to be stupid or if we are going to get their pussy. Intelligence is a turn on for women, so be alert. Every time you walk away from a situation and you didn't get what you wanted, think about it and see if you can figure out where you went wrong and do it differently the next time.

"Do you have a plan?" -- She wants to know that you want to fuck and what your plan your plans are…the way you want it to go down…and the logistics of it. Where, when, how…not necessarily how you want to have sex with her, but where & when…the location you want to do it at, the sequence of events (I'll pick you up here, we'll do this, then we will go here and have sex…).

"Do you have any questions for me?" -- She is giving you a chance to ask her if she wants to have sex… She may have just grilled you or put you through a line of intense questioning or whatever, and you have passed her test and now she is giving you a chance to get what you want… Go ahead and ask her for it!

"Thanks for Coming!" -- I've heard this a few times before it dawned on me that the women literally meant, "Cumming!" They may say this when you first get there or they may say it when you leave, or in response to your follow-up text that you always send immediately after you leave their sight when the date is over… Your immediate response to this comment is again, "You wanna come over?" or "Wanna have some fun?"

THE 2 MOST IMPORTANT QUESTIONS
TO GET SEX

"Wanna Come Over?" &
"Wanna Have Sex?"

Given the understanding that all women want sex and when she is ready for it, she is ready for it, and when she is ready for it, then you need to take her somewhere that you can get it on; hence the question, "Wanna come over?" This question will pretty much tell her what's up and what your intentions are... This question alone may be enough to get her to come over and fuck you.

Some women want a little more clarification than that and may want to test your confidence and see if you have the balls to specifically ask for what you really want; therefore, the question, "Do you wanna have sex?" or just, "Wanna have sex?"

These two questions are specifically meant to be asked together, back to back. You ask, "Wanna come over?" Then you wait for her to give her response, and then you ask your next question, "Wanna have sex?" You can either do this in person or you can do it on the phone or in a text-message. In person, of course, is usually the best, depending on the situation. Sometimes, you will only have a chance in person and if you don't ask then, that may be your last chance. If you have a chance on text-message then you can do that too, which in certain circumstances may be more appropriate; like if you were with her somewhere where it would have been extremely awkward for her because of who else was around...

"Sex," can mean different things for different people. This is why sometimes, it is just best to be specific about it and ask for "Sex." Sometimes, you may use the word, "Fun," as in, "Do you wanna have some fun?" This can be taken different ways, depending on the woman. Some women may associate sex with fun and some may not necessarily. For some, they may only have sex with someone that they are considering having a relationship with and may take it more seriously, while others may not care and can call it fun because they enjoy it so much, regardless of any relationship.

If you come across a woman that will only have sex with someone that she is considering a relationship with and you say, "Wanna have some fun?" She may think that you just want to use her for sex and don't want anything else. This is why, it is better to just straight up ask her if she wants to have "Sex."

After you ask your first question, "You wanna come over?" She may offer some resistance to you, which is usually the case. She might say that she can't, that she has something else to do…or get a little more serious and say that she just met you… You have to at least try to push through this resistance. That's why you ask the second follow-up question, "Do you wanna have sex?"

It clarifies that you know what you want and you are not afraid to ask for it. It also shows that you are not afraid of a little resistance and that you are not going to let her intimidate you into backing down and not asking. Sometimes with getting sex fast, if you ask the first question, "Wanna come over?" But you don't ask the second question, "Wanna have sex?" Then she may not give you another chance and that's just the way that it goes sometimes.

You have to make a choice of whether you are going to go the traditional route of being the nice guy and pursuing a relationship, or sex slowly, or you are just going to go straight for it. This book is about going straight for it.

There is always a risk to that though. If you decide to go the fast sex route, then you have to be willing to take the chance of completely blowing your opportunity with her very quickly. If it doesn't go the way that you want and you don't get sex right away, then you probably won't get anything from her. You just have to keep moving and meeting new women until you do get one that wants it.

On the other side of the coin, I'm sure we are all aware of the old traditional nice guy route of asking a woman out to dinner and maybe dating her for a while, hoping that sex will happen sometime... Well, this book is not about that. It's not about wasting your time, effort and resources like that. It's simply about going straight for the jugular and getting what you want now.

Naturally, nobody wants to wait for what they want. If you can get it now, you get it now and this is how I discovered fast sex. I would see a woman that I was attracted to and instantly know that I wanted to have sex with her. I thought, why should I wait and waste my time and spend a bunch of money and effort... Why can't I just go straight for it? Then I started spotting little clues in women's behavior that told me that something more was possible and I just kept following those leads to see where they led and they led me to these understandings.

If there is something that you want, then just go straight for it and stop wasting your time. Life is too short to waste waiting. If she is not ready, then there will be someone else who is. Life is designed this way. If you have a desire, then there is always a way to get it. So, go for it and don't give up until you get it!

TEXTING
(a Powerful Tool)

Texting is an awesome way to do some easy gaming, which takes a lot of the awkwardness out of talking, having awkward silences, running out of things to say, not knowing what to say and not having enough time to think of the right things to say and saying the wrong things because of it. It also eliminates having to worry about using the wrong tone voice. All of which, can instantly blow your opportunities with women. Texting gives you much more of a chance to get it right. Most women these days are into texting and actually prefer texting for all of the above reasons. It also allows them to respond when it is convenient for them. Instead of having to interrupt what they are doing, they can simply respond when they have a fee moment and allows you to continue the conversation for as long as you wish, which will also keep you on her mind. Also, you can say things that may be awkward in person or in public, for both you and her. Texts can also be very brief which allows you to get straight to the point and send them at times when a phone call may be inappropriate or too risky to make. All in all, texting is a great way to communicate and stay in touch.

Text Key Phrases & Symbols

All the previous keywords & phrases also apply to texting. In addition, the following are also helpful to understand:

:)   The smiley face is one of the biggest and most clear text signs that a woman will give you if she wants to have sex. I'm not saying that it always means that, just as with any other word or phrase, but this is very common if she is in the mood. So pay attention! If she gives you the smiley face, then it couldn't hurt to ask her if she wants to "Come over…"

;)   Another variation on the smiley face is the smiley face with a wink, using the semi-colon. This one is even more suggestive. It's like saying, "Hint, Hint." Get it? For instance, if a woman texted you, "Can I get that massage? ;)" Then obviously, she is saying that she wants sex. Or if she texts, "I just got off work ;)" then she is hinting that she wants to see you… When she adds the smile with a wink, that means that she wants a little more than what she is saying with words and that she wants you to take it to the next level. A plain smiley face can mean the same thing but the winky smile is making it that much more obvious.

... Dot, dot, dot, of course, means, etc, etc. Or "And so on," which means that she wants things to keep moving forward or progressing. This is usually also a good sign, as long as she's saying something that you like. For example, if she texts, "Have a good day ... " that is a good sign because she is most likely hinting that she wants to see you that day...

! The exclamation point emphasizes something. With flirtatious texts, it can mean much more. A lot of women hold back from using exclamation points "!" unless they are really trying to give you a hint about something. It's just about the same as them using "..." Each additional exclamation point she uses in a row increases the meaning and makes it much more impactful. If she texts, "See you soon!!!" Then she is *really* interested in seeing you!

LOL or **lol** Meaning, "Laugh out loud." This is a good one to use to lighten the mood. If you texted, "Wanna have some fun? lol" that makes it flirtier and gives her an obvious flirtatious hint that you want to have sex... If you can get her laughing and she is using "lol" too, that's good. It means that she wants to be playful with you. The more playful she is, the more likely she will want to have sex with you.

??? Sometimes women will put three question marks after a question. This is usually to test you and see if you are confident enough to say what you really want. It's usually a trick question. They are putting more emphasis on it to try to intimidate you, so that you think you have to answer it correctly. The correct answer is to say what you really want!

Ttyl or **ttyl** Talk to you later. If you can't connect with a woman right then and she doesn't want to commit to any plans, then just text, "Ok. ttyl" then hit her up another time.

Approaches
(it all starts here)

I will give you a few different scenarios so you can see how it works depending on how she responds... In general, I have a pretty flat out direct and simple approach. It goes something like this:

Scenario 1
(Approach, Get Her Number & Follow-Up)

You: "Hi, my name is _____. I thought you looked really cute and I just wanted to come and say, Hi."

Her: "Oh, Hi!"

This creates an opening. You can throw her another compliment, like compliment her on something she is wearing or ask her some curious question you have and start a conversation or just go straight on to the following lines:

You: "What's your name?"

Her: "My name is Jenny."

You: "Hi, Jenny. I'm _____."

Then you can stick out your hand and give her a nice soft handshake. I know that everyone says you should give a firm handshake, but to me, this is too business-like. This is something that you can play with and see what works best for you. I like to feel a woman's softness. I feel it is more sensual. I focus more on the energy I feel when I touch a woman and I can feel that better if I relax my hand.

You: "I was just wondering if you would join me for some coffee?"

Her: "Actually, I'm kind of busy right now..."

You: "Can I get your number?"

Her: "Ok, sure."

Whip out your cell phone and put her number in or get out a pen and paper if you don't have a cell phone with you. In general, it is always good to have your cell phone with you if at all possible, as I will show you how to follow-up with an immediate text message, which I highly recommend and will explain why shortly. Usually, I will just type her number in as she tells it to me, just like I'm going to call her and then I hit 'send' or 'call' and then hang up. This way, her number is in my phone and it's quick and easy and doesn't create any awkwardness by taking too long. I'll enter her name and a description after I leave. Every second and part of your interaction with a new woman is critical and any little thing may blow it, so I like to make it quick and easy.

You: "It was good meeting you! I'll talk to you soon."

Her: "Bye!"

This is the most common scenario, because she is most likely busy doing something at the moment, so you grab her number and follow up. (More on how to follow-up later in this section).

Another thing I discovered is that it's good to have a standard approach, with a few standard key questions lined up ready to ask, because it gives you more ammo to push through her resistance with. As I said earlier, she will not usually say yes on your 1st try. For example, if you start off with your standard approach:

"Hi, my name is _____. I just thought you looked really cute and wanted to come and say, Hi."

And then you ask her out to coffee…

This gives her something to say, "No," to. Then you have your next question ready to go:

"Can I get your get your number?"

She may give you her number or she may, again, say, "No."

If she says, "No," then you can ask her if she wants to be, "Friends."

If she says, "No," to this then that is usually it, but at least you have your approach and 3 standard key questions lined up and ready to go. If she says, "No," to the first or second question, then you still have another question that she may change her mind and say, "Yes," to. You see, sometimes she just wants to see that you are really trying and that you really want her and aren't going to give up too easily. It took me a while to figure this out at first. When I first began, I would hear the first, "No," and that would be it. I would give up and walk away. Then I started trying to persist a little and found that on the second or third question, she would, a lot of times, say "Yes," and I just started figuring out each next step along the way. Something deep down in me, and her expressions & body language, were telling me that more was possible.

Scenario 2
(Approach & Get an Instant Date)

You: "Hi, my name is _____. I thought you looked really cute and I just wanted to come and say, Hi."

Her: "Oh, Hi!"

You: "What's your name?"

Her: "My name is Jenny."

You: "Hi, Jenny. I'm _____."

Shake hands

You: "I was just wondering if you would join me for some coffee?"

Her: "Right now?"

You: "mm-hmm, yah."

Her: "Ok"

Then you can pick the closest coffee shop or can even ask her if she wants to go to a bar and get a drink. Or you can go to a restaurant that has a bar too and sit at the bar or wherever. I prefer sitting at a bar because you can sit right next to her and touch her when you are talking to her. Touching can greatly increase your odds of getting sex when done right. This is a great scenario if you meet in a shopping mall because you can just walk with her to the coffee shop or bar in the mall. (You will be given more information on how to interact on a date in the Date section.)

Scenario 3
(Approach & Join Her)

This approach is if you are at, say, a coffee shop, fast food restaurant, or somewhere where she is sitting by herself…

You: "Hi, my name is _____. I thought you looked really cute and I just wanted to come and say, Hi."

Her: "Oh, Hi!"

You: "Can I join you?"

Her: "Sure!"

Sit down and join her.

You: "What's your name?"

Her: "My name is Jenny."

You: "Hi, Jenny. I'm _____."

Shake her hand. You can then throw her another compliment, like compliment her on something she is wearing, or ask her some curious question you have and start a conversation...

You will be given more information on how to interact in the *Dates* section.

Scenario 4
(Approach & Get Sex)

You: "Hi, my name is _____. I thought you looked really cute and I just wanted to come and say, Hi."

Her: "Oh, Hi!"

You: "What's your name?"

Her: "My name is Jenny."

You: "Hi, Jenny. I'm _____."

Shake hands

You: "I was just wondering if you would join me for some coffee?"

Her: "I'm in a relationship."

You: "You wanna be friends?"

(Some women will really perk up and smile when you ask them this and you will get a very clear sign that she is available for sex. Be confident & follow through.)

Her: "Sure!"

You: "You wanna come over?"

(If she answers, "Ok" then you can skip the following lines.)

Her: "Come over?"

You: "You wanna have some fun?" (Smile, if you can naturally.)

Her: "Ok!"

Have her follow you to your place and have some fun! :)

Immediate Follow-Up Text Message
After Getting Her Number

You always want to make sure, as often as possible, to have your cell phone with you. This way, when you meet a woman you can immediately put her number in your phone as you are talking to her. Then you can follow-up with an immediate text message…

Cell phones and texting are an essential part of *getting sex fast*! As soon as you get a woman's number and walk away from her, you want to send her an immediate follow-up text message. The reason for this is because your interaction with her may have got her turned on and thinking about sex. There is nothing more exciting than the initial thrill of having sex with someone new. The mystery, the intrigue…plus, you haven't yet got on her bad side yet or upset her in any way…so you are still a fresh fantasy for her. For all she knows, you might be the perfect one that she's been waiting for her whole life. You want to take immediate advantage of this state in a woman's mind because you will never again have that chance with her. This is why fast sex works and what it is all about…the initial excitement, the rush, the thrill…the SEX!!!

As soon as you get her number and walk away, send her an immediate follow-up text message. Here are some examples of text messages that I use:

1) "Good meeting you, Jenny! Have a good day. (your name)"

2) "Good meeting you, Jenny! See you soon. :) (your name)"

3) "Good meeting you! Talk to you soon. (your name)"

Another good reason to send an immediate follow-up text is that you give her your name and number right away, that way she'll know who it is when you contact her again. Also, it establishes an immediate connection. Instead of you waiting a day or two to contact her and maybe she has changed her mind since then and decides to brush you off… She will feel more connection and obligation to respond to you since you have already contacted her before.

The main reason, though, of the immediate follow-up text is the booty call. If she responds immediately or, say, within 5 minutes, then there is a really good chance that she wants sex right now, or very soon! It's a test to see how interested she is, it also depends on how she responds. Here are some good examples of possible responses that may indicate that she wants sex:

1) "Good meeting you too! Have a good day!!! :)"

2) "See you soon!!!"

3) "You too!!! See you soon …"

If you get an immediate response with a very positive vibe, such as in the previous examples, then definitely respond back immediately with:

"You wanna come over? :)" or "Wanna have some fun?"

If she responds back and asks where you live?

Then text her your address or wherever you plan on meeting her and wait for her to respond.

If she asks what you have in mind or something to that effect, then text:

"Wanna have sex? :)"

She may offer some resistance, as a test, as most women do. She may text something like:

1) "I can't. I have an appointment."

2) "I'm driving."

3) "Next time!"

4) "It was good meeting you but I have to be somewhere. Talk to you later."

In most cases, women will offer some kind of resistance because they don't want to seem too easy. It is your job to push through this and show them that you have some balls and that you know what you want! Since she responded immediately to your text, she probably wants it. If she did not want it right then, she probably would have either, not responded so quickly and maybe waited an hour or more, or she may not have responded at all and waited for you to contact her again later. Since she did respond right away, I would push through and give it a shot at least.

After she responds with resistance, you text back:

"Wanna have sex? :)"

Wait for her response... If she asks where you live, text her your address and wait for her to respond. If she sounds offended, you can text something like one of the following:

1) "How about a game of cards?"

2) "Want to listen to some music and talk?"

3) "Wanna watch a movie?"

Any reason to get her to come over to your place is fine. If she goes for it and comes over, then most likely she wants sex, otherwise she would not come over after you asked her to have sex. Again, she may just not want to seem that easy, so she wants another reason to come over...

After Dates
(follow-up)

Same thing after having a date with a woman, you want to send her an immediate follow-up text as soon as you get out of her sight, within the first minute or two if you can; but no later than 5 minutes. If for some reason you forget to, then go ahead and send it as soon as you remember. I usually send the following:

"Good seeing you!"

See how she responds. If she responds right away with a positive vibe, then there is a good possibility that she may want to come over and have sex.

Follow up with, "Wanna come over? :)" …

And continue the same as in the previous section…

Next Day Call
(keep going)

A lot of women don't respond to the Immediate Follow-Up Text. In fact, most don't, but it's definitely worth a shot because if they're ready to go. then they are ready to go and you don't want to miss that opportunity as it could always be your last.

That being said, if they don't respond then I will give them a call the next day. The ideal time would probably be between 8 to 9 pm since most women will be home relaxing by that time. Depending on her situation though, and whether she is working during the day or not, the late morning or middle of the day could be good too, say, anywhere between 10 am and 2 pm. That way, if she is free then you could possibly meet for coffee right then or set up a date for when she gets off work that evening. It also depends on when you are free to make a call and receive one back from her in case she doesn't answer but gets your message.

My basic routine goes something like this, if she answers, you say:

"Hi, Jenny it's _____ from yesterday at the mall. How are you?"

Her: "Oh, Hi! I'm good. How are you?"

You: "I'm good. I was just wondering if you want to grab some coffee with me?"

Her: "Ok, sure."

You: "How about we meet at the coffee shop at the mall at 3?"

Her: "Ok, sounds good!"

You: "I'll see you then!"

If right then is not good for her and she is interested, she will, most likely, let you know when a good time for her is. You can also discuss where you would like to meet, but in general, being the man, she most likely wants you to lead and make the suggestions about where to go, etc. She should let you know what time she is free, if she is not free right then. But you make the initial suggestion as to what time and where... If she says she is busy and does not suggest a time that she is available, then you can ask her when she is free. If she will not commit to a time and says that she is too busy right now, then just say:

"Ok. I'll talk to you later. Have a good day!"

With a smile on your face and see how she responds.

If she responds really positively and says,

"You too!" in kind of a flirtatious, happy way, then you can ask her to "Come over" right then. See how she responds and continue in the way described in *Immediate Follow-Up Texts*, but with your voice on the phone.

If she doesn't seem that friendly, you can just say, "Ok, have a good day," and just leave it at that for now and then hit her up in a few days with a late night booty text; which I will describe in the next section, or you can send her an immediate text right then and see how she responds.

If you decide to send her an immediate follow-up text, you can say something like:

"Good talking to you!" And leave it at that.

If she responds positively to it, then you can continue as in the *Immediate Follow-Up Texts* section…

If she doesn't answer the phone, and a voicemail comes on, then I will leave the following message:

"Hi Jenny, it's _____ from the mall yesterday! Just wondering if you want to grab some coffee with me? Give me a call, my number is _____. Hope you're having a great day! Bye!"

(If you say it with a smile, it will sound more appealing and she will hear it in your voice).

Leave it at that and see if she responds. If not, you can hit her up with a late night booty text in a few days as described in the next section.

Booty Calls / Texts
(catch her when she's in the mood)

Booty calls are those late night calls or texts that you make to her to see if she is in the mood for a little fun… This is the ideal time for a lot of women because during the day they may be busy with work, school, shopping or other activities. And this is the time that she is most likely relaxing, not doing much of anything, maybe lying in bed and maybe even thinking about sex… So it's the perfect time to hit her up. Also, it's a good time because it is late and after dark and most other people are asleep, so she doesn't have to worry much about anyone seeing her come over and worrying about her reputation…

I usually use this as a last resort, if she didn't respond to my *immediate follow-up text* or to my *next day call*. However, I will usually wait until 3 or 4 days after my Next Day Call.

Typically booty calls are done between the hours of 10 pm & 2 am. Use a little psychology with this to determine how late you want to do it. Think about the kind of woman she is: how old is she? Does she work in the morning? Does she go to school? What's her schedule like? Is she a more conservative type or is she more flirtatious? Is it a Friday or Saturday night where she can most likely stay up later? I would say though, that probably the main determining factor is her age. Older women above 40 years old, you probably want to hit them up a little earlier, say between, 9 & 11 pm since they don't have quite as much energy as younger women. For younger women under 40, if it's a weeknight, probably between 11 pm & Midnight and if it's a Friday or Saturday night, between Midnight & 2 am. Again, play around with it and find out what works best for you and the women you are approaching.

For late night booty calls, I prefer text-messaging. This is a tricky situation…it is late at night and you don't always know what her situation is. You don't know whether she is in a relationship, if she lives with anyone…so, text messaging is a lot simpler, gets the message across and is straight to the point. It also reduces the risk of you messing things up by saying the wrong things or using the wrong tone of voice, etc… She could also be sleeping and a ringing phone may piss her off more than a one-time ring from a text-message.

I prefer using one of these simple phrases when I send a late night booty text:

1) "How are you?"

2) "What are you doing?"

3) "What are you up to?"

You could also use any one of these with a smiley face at the end if you want to. Just keep experimenting and trying different things to see what works for you and take note of the responses you get.

If they respond, then text them back and ask if they want to come over: "Wanna come over? :)"

Proceed as in the *Immediate Follow-Up Text* section...and beware, most likely she will give you some form of resistance, so be prepared to push through it and go for what you want! Also, being in a flirty, playful state of mind may help to loosen her up. After all, it is about, "Having Fun!" :)

Here are some examples of late night booty texts:

Scenario 1

(10:33 pm, weeknight)

You: "What are you doing?"

Her: "At the gym. Done working out." (10:40 pm)

You: "Wanna come over? :)" (10:44 pm)

Her: "I'm driving now. Can't text. Have to get up early for meeting tomorrow. Have a good night!" (11:33 pm)

You: "Wanna have sex? :)" (12:33)

Her: "Where do you live?" (12:34)

You: "(Your address)" (12:35)

Her: "Ok :)" (12:36)

Her: "Be there in 30 min" (12:37)

You: "K. See u then :)" (12:38)

Notice how at 11:33 she gives resistance in the form of words. The trap, for most men, is that they are more logical/left-brained and place too much focus on words instead of other signs. Notice the clues that she is interested: she responded at exactly 11:33, exactly 1 hour after you sent your 1st text at 10:33 AND the Exclamation point at the end of, "Have a good night!" You see, women do this stuff all the time, they will tell us with their words, "No," but with other signs, they will say an astounding, "Yes!" You have to listen to the other signs. Even more-so, you have to listen to yourself!!! You have to know what you want and go for it anyways!!! No matter what the other signs are telling you! The universe, including women will always test you to see if you want it bad enough!!! Well, do you???

Scenario 2

(11:01 pm, weeknight)

You: "How are you?"

Her: "I'm good & u?"

You: "I'm good. You wanna come over? :)"

Her: "It's been a long day. I'm tired." (Resistance)

You: "Wanna have sex? :)"

Her: "I don't think my boyfriend would like that" (Resistance)

You: "Just friends, right? :)"

Her: "Are you sure? friends without sex???"
(Trick question)

You: "Ok, sex... lol"

No response

You: "You want to come?"

Her: "Just friends right?" (Caution)

You: "Yep"

Her: "Ok, where do you live?"

You: "(Your address)"

Her: "Who do you live with?" (Caution)

You: "By myself"

Her: "K. See u in a little bit..."

A lot of times, I send my texts at a time when there is multiple of the same digits in a row (ex: 11:01, 11:33, 12:22…), just for the fun of it. I'll explain a little about this in the next section. Immediately after she responds to your first text, you ask, "Wanna come over?" She then responds with some resistance, then you shoot the next big question off, "Wanna have sex?" Then she comes across with even more resistance. Anytime they use their relationship as resistance, you make clear that it's just, "Friends." Then she gives you a trick question to see if you are going to be a dumb-ass and say yes. If you say yes to this, then kiss your chances of sleeping with her good-bye. She can use this against you in the future if you try to bring up having sex again. This is another reason that text messaging is beautiful because it gives you time to think of the best response. You will make mistakes here and there and blow chances, but this is how you learn and improve. Believe me, you are far better off for reading this stuff than I ever was, having to learn it for myself. You will be much further ahead for it.

Then you respond with humor to her trick question, reaffirming that yes, you want sex. She does too, but any slip-ups could blow your chances. If so, you just have to move on to the next. Some women will give you multiple chances, as I will explain later. The beautiful thing is though, once your game is sharpened, you will get women left and right if you want to.

After you reaffirm that you want sex, she does not respond because she doesn't want to make it too easy for you. You just have to know what you want and keep moving forward and she will either give it to you or she won't, but you just keep moving…

After no response from her, you use a clever double-meaning to ask again if she wants to come over, "You want to come?" This also insinuates having sex, which can turn her on and motivate her to come over. She then uses caution to make sure that the sex is just for fun and nothing serious, by confirming that you are just friends again. She is already in a relationship and doesn't want to change that, so she wants your agreement. After your confirmation, she then says Ok. Then she throws out one more question of caution, "Who do you live with?" Some women will only come over if you live alone. They are very cautious with their reputation and don't want anyone else knowing about what's going on. They don't want to run in to anyone else unexpectedly that may compromise their discretion.

The smart thing to say is that you live alone. Let's say you live with some roommates in a house…just be creative and frame it as a studio apartment and say that you have a, "Studio." Whatever the case, just make it sound like you live alone, or else she may not come over and you will not get laid.

Scenario 3

(11:33 pm, weeknight)

You: "What are you up to?"

Her: "Reading"

You: "Wanna come over?"

Her: "What are you thinking???"   (Test)

You: "Just a little fun before bed... lol ;)"

Her: "Hmmm..."

Her: "Have to get up early tmr"   (Resistance)

You: "Wanna have sex?"

No response   (Resistance)

You: "It'll help you sleep better, I promise! ;)" (Humor)

Her: "Hahaha"

Her: "Where do you live?"

You: "(Your address)"

Her: "Well, ok. Just for a little bit though..."

Her: "So this is going to help me sleep better huh?"

You: "I promise"

Her: "Ok, see u! ;)"

Notice, after you asked your first big question, "Wanna come over?" She tests you by asking, "What are you thinking???" To some newbies who are a little insecure and not sure of themselves, you might think that she is being critical, and get scared and back down. Again, you have to know what you want and push through your fear and go for it anyways and ask your next big question in one way or another. If you want Sex, or whatever it is that you want in life, then you have to have the balls to ask for it!!! Women will always test you, so ask for what you REALLY want!!!

Then, of course, she again offers her resistance by making an excuse...which, as usual, they always do, to see if you really know what you want and how badly you want it. She offers more resistance after your next big question, by not responding. You push through this time by using a little humor. Humor is a great way to loosen women up. If you can make them laugh enough, you can have sex with them. Laughter has a way of opening people up and helping them to let go.

Sometimes, women will not always respond right then and there to the booty text. If they get back to you at a later time, are positive and still want to see you, then that means they want sex too. Otherwise, they wouldn't get back to you. They may get back to you at a time that is more convenient for them. Then just proceed and keep going for it. You will have to play it by ear and go with their flow, but keep going... Sometimes, you have to take 2 steps forward and 1 step backwards, otherwise it may be too fast for them. It all depends on the woman.

Text Games
(women love to play, play along)

Some women play, what I call, "Text Games." I discovered this by observing the patterns of when some women texted me. I started noticing that a lot of women would text me at times like: 1:11, 2:22, 3:33, or 11:33, 11:44, 11:55… Then I started trying this at times. I would text her at 1:11 and she would text me back at 2:22…or I would text her at 11:33 and she would text me at 11:44. Then I noticed sometimes she would text me at 3:32 and I realized that she wanted me to text her back at 3:33… I realized that women sometimes use these as, "Windows of opportunity," for us men.

Some women also play the game of giving you, 1 minute, to respond and if you don't respond within that minute, you don't get any. Say you text her at 3:11 with, "Wanna come over?" She may text you back at 3:32 with, "Busy right now…" Don't just pay attention to the words she's saying, look at the other clues she is giving you: it is 3:32 (almost 3:33) and the end of her text was, "…" meaning, *and so on*, meaning, *your move*… As soon as you get a text from her, look at the time. Since you know now that women play the resistance game and it is now 3:32 and she just responded to your question with resistance, it is now perfect time to hit her with your next question at 3:33, "Wanna have sex? :)"

Just as in person with women, time is of the essence with text messaging. As the say, "Time waits for no one," and neither do women.

So, check it out, play with it, explore and see what new patterns and observations you can spot that women are using, so you can play along with them and use it to your advantage. They will see that you are intelligent, observant and understand what is going on and it will score you points in their eyes and between their legs…

1 Week
(sequence)

I have a normal routine that I go through when I meet a woman I want to have sex with. So far, you have the mind-set, key phrases, approaches, immediate follow-up texts, next day call, & booty call/text. Now, I will show you how to plan and space everything out so you can juggle all the new women that you will be meeting.

It's good to get a weekly planner that shows the whole week, all 7 days, in one glance and has time slots. When I meet a new woman, I will jot down in the planner when I met her and did my immediate follow-up text. If she did not respond, I will write down when I plan to give her the next day call. If she does not respond to that, I will schedule 2 to 4 days ahead and write down what day, time and what I want to say in my booty text to her.

It is good to have it all scheduled out and execute things as planned. That way you keep track of what you are doing with each woman, experiment with time patterns and the spacing of your actions. Keep improving on it, develop your own system and see what works best for you. This way also, you don't forget to execute your next moves because you look in your planner everyday and jot down on a piece of paper what you are going to do that day and at what time and carry it with you so you remember.

As you keep meeting women, ad them to your planner with what you have done so far and your following planned actions. This way you can make sense out of it all and juggle them instead of being confused as to which one you are going to contact at which time...

For instance, say you go shopping on Friday afternoon at a few different stores. You meet Nancy at store 1. You do your immediate follow-up text to her. She doesn't respond. You meet Sue at store 2. She responds to your immediate text but is not available that day. At store 3, you meet Tina and she does not respond to your immediate follow-up text and at store 4, you meet Julie, who decides to be friends with you and come over right then.

The next day, Saturday around noon, you text Sue because she did respond to your immediate follow-up text, so you know she is ok with texting and seemed interested but was busy. The text interaction goes like this:

You: "How are you?"

Her: "I'm good & u?"

You: "I'm good. You wanna grab some coffee?"

Her: "I would but I'm busy today"

You: "When's good for you?"

Her: "I'll let you know"

You: "K. ttyl"

Since she didn't want to commit to anything, I will schedule a booty text to her for Tuesday night around 11 pm. If they don't show enough interest to commit to anything then there are really only 2 options: you can either let it go and not contact her anymore or you can give it one last shot with a late night booty text. You may as well give it one last shot, instead of just letting it go. Sometimes, this is just what they are looking for.

A lot of times, this is the case, where she just wants sex. Otherwise, she would have taken you up on your offer to have coffee, but since she doesn't show any interest in getting to know you, then obviously she is not looking for a relationship, but she may just want sex. After all, there is a reason that she gave you her number to begin with; otherwise, she would have just blown you off or ignored you all together when she met you.

However, before you make that last late night booty text, you want to go through the previous routine to make it look like you are a normal guy and not like you only want sex. Since she has not reciprocated, then there is nothing wrong with giving it one last shot and seeing if she wants to have sex.

Since Sue didn't want to get together today, you do your next day voice calls to the other 2 women that did not respond to your immediate follow-up texts. You make your 1st call to Nancy. She doesn't answer, so you leave the following message:

"Hi Nancy, it's _____ from the store yesterday, just seeing if you wanna grab some coffee with me. Give me a call. My number is _____. Hope you're having a good day!"

Give it an hour or so to see if she responds before making your next call to Tina. Ok, so Nancy doesn't respond and you make your next call to Tina. She answers and the conversation goes like this:

Her: "Hello"

You: "Hi Tina, it's _____ from yesterday at the store. How are you?"

Her: "Oh, Hi! I'm good and you?"

You: "I'm good. I was just wondering if you want to join me for some coffee?"

Her: "Sure. That sounds good. I'm kind of in the middle of something right now, but how about around 7?"

You: "Ok, sure, how about Rick's Café, at the mall where we met?"

Her: "Sure. That sounds good. I'll see you then!"

You: "Ok, see you then!"

It is always good to call from the same phone that you sent your immediate follow-up text from when you first met her. That way she recognizes the number and knows it's you and will be more likely to answer if she's interested. A lot of women will not answer the phone if they don't recognize the number and it is more likely that she will agree to meet you if you actually talk to her versus leaving her a message.

So, Nancy, your 1st next day call never gets back to you and you schedule a late night booty text to her for Wednesday around 11 pm and Tuesday you have your late night booty text scheduled for Sue.

Do you see how it works? You always do your immediate follow-up text just after you meet them to see if they are either interested in hooking up right then or to at least gauge their level of interest to determine your next move. If they do not respond, you schedule your next day voice call to them. If they do not respond to that, then you schedule their late night booty text from 2 to 4 days later.

I recommend doing your late night booty texts on weeknights as a lot of attractive women may already have previous plans on Friday or Saturday night, but you can play with that. It is ideal if you only schedule 1 booty text per weeknight. If you are meeting a lot of women, then you may need to schedule more than 1 per night so that you don't wait too long to booty text them. Since this is your last resort because they haven't responded favorably to your previous contacts, there is at least a 50% chance that they won't respond to this one. If you have to stagger more than one on the same night then you can do that. Say you have 2 booty texts that you want to do that night, maybe text one at around 10:30, see if she responds, if not, you can do the other one around 11:30 or Midnight.

If you start approaching women everywhere you go, then you will start meeting a lot of women and they will start to accumulate and you will have to juggle them. That's why it is smart to have a planner and to schedule your future contacts with each one, so that you can space them out smoothly and plan it so that you don't forget any important steps.

Sometimes Several Chances
(don't give up)

A lot of times, some women will only give you one chance at their pussy and others may give you several chances. However, if you miss one opportunity, you may have to wait a while for another chance with her. You may get 2 or 3 chances within 1 week with her but then if you miss those and she is no longer responding to your calls or text messages, then I highly recommend letting it go for a while.

If you really don't care and are not that interested in her, then you can just let it go altogether. If you are very attracted to her, then just let it go for a while and maybe contact her in 2 to 4 weeks. It really all depends on the interactions that you have had with her and how they went. Sometimes, there is a strong attraction between you both, but you just blew your chances because you were unaware at the moment. This happens a lot, especially at first. Life is a mystery and it's always challenging us. I would say that seducing woman can be one of the most challenging things there is, but it is also one of the most interesting, worthwhile and exciting things there is too. Women are mysterious and you never really know how it is going to go with them. You will always learn something new all the time.

If you blow a few chances with her and she is not responding to you anymore, you can just let it go altogether or you can wait a while and give it another try. The whole idea is to let her wonder about you, miss you and think that maybe that was the last time she will hear from you. Then out of the blue, you surprise her and contact her.

Remember too, where you were with her, meaning how far you got with her. Like say you did a late night booty text and she was responding favorably and you just blew it by making the wrong move and she stopped responding. Well, after you take a break and give it another try, you can most likely start where you left off. You don't have to start at the beginning again. You may want to take one step backwards from where you were and start there... It just depends, you have to use a little bit of your own intuition and kind of feel where it is that you would like to start off or where you think would be a good place.

While you are taking that break from her, certain feelings or ideas may cross your mind and you may have an intuition that gives you an insight as to how you should start it off with her the next time. Listen to those intuitions, as everything is connected and those thoughts and feelings that are urging you to re-connect with her are actually part of the same energy that she is connected to. If you have an urge to re-connect with her, then there is a really good possibility that she would like to re-connect with you as well. It's all connected. Your feelings and desires are God's feelings and desires for you and you are meant to act on them and make them happen. We are not given a desire without the ability to fulfill that desire. Our desires are seeds that God planted within us that are meant to lead us to our purpose and destiny, so express your desires and live the life you were meant to live. You were meant to be happy and fulfilled. Trust in that and watch it work wonders in your life.

DATES
(there's nothing like being face to face)

If you didn't get sex with her when you met her and you did your immediate follow-up text and didn't get sex right then or later as a result of it, then you will most likely have to meet her somewhere and go on a date. I suggest something simple where you don't have to spend much time or money. The last thing you want is to waste much time, effort or money on her if you don't know that you will get what you want in return. I'd say, once you are sleeping with her and if you really like her, then fine, do whatever you want. If you over-invest in her and nothing happens, you will just feel like a frustrated chump that's been taken advantage. This is why I suggest coffee or something very simple that doesn't cost much and won't take much of your time or be too awkward if things don't go well.

Another thing is, if you asked her to come over or for sex in any of your previous interactions and she said no, but is still willing to go on a date with you, then obviously she is interested in sex. Otherwise, she wouldn't see you again after knowing what you want.

Coffee / Drink
(a cheap, simple place to meet)

I highly suggest that for a 1st date, you just meet her for something simple like coffee or a drink of some kind, something where you just grab the drink in a to-go cup. That way, you have already paid for it and if things don't go well, then you can just take it and leave. It also allows more flexibility. Say, things go well and she asks you where you live and you ask her to come over and she says yes...then you can just leave right away while the vibe is good. The last thing you want is to get a yes from her, and then because things are taking too long to leave and get on your way, she changes her mind. Women are very fickle and can change their mind in a second. You never really know how it is going to go, that's why I suggest something simple where you can just get up and go when you need to.

The last thing you want is to get stuck in the middle of a big dinner with her if things aren't going well and have to finish and pay and have an awkward time. Not to mention, wasting your money. With fast sex, things can move very rapidly. If you ask a key question or get a signal from her and she says yes, then you need to be able to leave right then.

A lot of times, she will give you a key signal, like asking where you live very soon, if not right away when you first get to the venue. You need to be able to respond immediately and ask her to come over and then be able to leave immediately if she says yes. Meeting for coffee or something that you've already paid for, allows you to do this.

The whole point is just to meet somewhere so that you can be face to face, talk, look for key signals from her, ask her the right questions and take her home when she says yes. Coffee…allows you to do that. For women who only want fast sex, a lot of times, this is all they will want to do anyways, because they don't want to waste time since they are not looking for a relationship.

Let Her Talk
(when she feels understood, she'll feel closer to you)

Something I learned from one of my good friends is that if you let someone talk, and just listen, without saying much or resisting with differing opinions…then that person will feel a lot closer to you emotionally. They will feel that you understand them and relieved that they could express themselves to you. Just look at them with an open expression and acknowledge them by nodding and agreeing with them.

There is so much conflict in life and I know that men, in particular, like to try to fix things or solve the problem. Women, on the other hand, just want someone to listen, so that they can express themselves. After they express themselves, they feel much better. If you let them express themselves, then maybe they will feel close enough to you to let you express yourself to them in the way that you want, if you know what I mean... If they feel close to you, then there is a good chance that they will want to have sex with you, because for women, a lot of having sex is about feeling a connection to the other person. If you let her talk and express herself, she will feel much more connected to you than if you talk a lot. In fact, women do not like a man that talks too much. They want a man that will listen and pay attention to them. It's a big turn-off for them if a man talks too much. If she wants sex, then she's going to have to feel a connection to you or at least feel that everything is going smoothly. It will only go smoothly if you don't stand in the way, by offering too many of your own opinions that conflict with hers.

If it doesn't seem like things are going very well and there is too much awkward silence, then ask her questions about herself to get her talking. As she is talking, pick out certain keywords or topics she mentions that strike you or sound interesting. When she stops talking, then ask her about them. If you keep doing this, you will be able to keep the conversation going and keep her talking. As she is talking, pay attention to any signs or clues she may be trying to give you that she wants sex.

Catch the Signs & Respond
(everything you need is here now)

There is a reason that she went out with you to begin with. Either she is just interested in sex or she is interested in a relationship too. My theory is, if you approached a random, complete stranger with my simple, straightforward approach and didn't really have much of a conversation and she gave you her number and went out with you, then she is probably a pretty open person, including sexually.

If she meets you for a date, the whole point is just to get her talking and listen for the clues that she is interested in you/sex and respond immediately to take advantage of it. If her body language is positive and she is interacting with you in a warm and friendly way, then she probably wants it. It is best, however, to wait for some signs from her and respond to them. That way, she will feel like it is her idea and that she wants it, rather than you forcing your manly agenda on her. This is why it is good if you can get her talking, because it gives you clues and signs to listen for, not to mention makes her feel closer to you emotionally.

One of the biggest signs that a woman is interested in you is that she is smiling. If she keeps smiling, then go ahead and lean over and give her a kiss. If she turns away or rejects it, then that's fine too, at least you tried and showed her that you are interested. Usually, if they are that friendly where they are smiling a lot, then even if she rejects the kiss right now, she will not be offended. She will be flattered that you tried. Or maybe she's just a little shy in public to kiss and that's fine too. I've met quite a few women like this.

If she's already in a relationship and just wants sex, then she will not want to kiss in public because she doesn't want anyone that she knows to see her. If this is the case, then it may be wise not to try kissing her in public... Have some respect for her and her relationship. If she continues to be friendly to you after you try to kiss her, then she is still interested. At this point, go ahead and ask her if she wants to come over... You may as well use that as an entry point and go for it. If she says no, then you can always follow-up with the second key question and ask her if she wants to have sex.

If she rejects it at this point, you can always hit her up later with an immediate follow-up text after the date and see how she responds. She may say no in person, but then hit on you after you send an immediate follow-up text and want to come over... Women do this a lot; they are testing to see if you are awake and will catch it. They will try to mess with your logic. Just because they said no before, doesn't mean that the next time they won't say yes. They like to play with this a lot. So, always, always, always send an immediate follow-up text anytime after you see them because it may be just what they are waiting for...

Also, another option is to hit them up that night with a booty text. If they say no in person and don't really flirt back with you when you send an immediate follow-up text, then go ahead and hit them up later that night with a booty text and see how they respond. They might be more in the mood just before bed anyways.

Always try to read between the lines with women. They are always playing with the way they communicate. They don't always communicate so directly with things like sex. Again, they don't want to feel like a slut so they will give you some hints and see if you catch them and bring it up, that way they can justify it by saying that *you* asked them.

Always be aware of key phrases, as I said before, when you first meet with her, a lot times she will ask where you live. She may ask, "What you are going to do after this?" She may say, "Thanks for coming," or "Have a good day!" These are all signs that you should ask her over. Also, something else I have noticed is that if she got coffee or some drink that she can hold in her hands, she may grasp it tightly with both hands and start kind of nervously squeezing or twisting her hands around it. If she does this, then ask her if she wants to have sex. They do this as a sign and they get nervous because, just as a man may get approach-anxiety before approaching a woman, women get nervous before they have sex with a new partner for the first time. So, if you notice that she is getting nervous, it may mean that this is a prime moment to ask her if she wants to have sex.

Notice the way she is dressed. Is it revealing? Is she showing cleavage? Is she wearing a short skirt or shorts that show off her legs? Tight clothes that accentuate her ass or boobs? Does her hair look really fancy? Did she put a lot of effort into the way that she looks? Does she smell nice? These are all really good signs that she wants you to notice her as a sexual being and may want sex.

Also, pay attention to her body language in general. Are her arms uncrossed and more open? Is she sticking her chest out so that you notice her boobs? Are her legs open? Or sticking her ass out? Smiling a lot as she looks at you? Playing with her hair? Leaning towards you? Does she laugh or smile a lot at the things you say, even though they may not be anything special or particularly funny? Laughter and smiling is definitely a good sign! All of these are good signs that she is interested. If she touches you, this is definitely a good sign! It probably means that she wants you to be touched by you...

If she compliments you, this is great sign that she is interested! Especially, if she compliments you on your looks or your body, then she is definitely interested in sex and you should go for it. Give her a compliment back about her looks or tell her she has a really sexy body. Ask her if she likes massages and tell her you give really good massages and see if she wants to come over for a massage... If she says no, smile and say, "How about sex?"

If she mentions sex in any way, shape or form, take that as a sign that she wants it. Even if she says she is not interested in sex, or that she doesn't understand the culture here and how fast people move sexually or whatever… She may just be pulling your leg and seeing if you are stupid enough to listen to her. This is, of course, if she mentions it on her own without you saying anything about it first. Even if you were to mention it, she still may be pulling your leg. You may turn around and make a move on her later and she may go for it or she may respond positively to a follow-up text or booty text later that night. You never know. Just don't take her too literally. Read into the things that she is saying. Sometimes, she just wants the subject of sex to come up and to get you thinking about it so that you will go for it…

Sometimes a woman may give you an opportunity in person, but then if you miss it and try to catch her later through texting or on the phone, she may blow you off. You never know. This is why you want to be as aware and alert as you can at each moment and pay attention to all the little clues and signs she is giving you and take advantage of them right away.

Middle of the Date
(do this)

If you hardly know a woman and she accepts a date with you, then that means she is interested, otherwise, she would not go out with a random stranger who just approached her out-of-the-blue. And if she accepted a date with a random stranger, then she probably wants sex and has already decided that if you play your cards right, you will get it. If this is the case, then sex is the whole point. So you want to make a point of it.

In the middle of your date, whether it is coffee, dinner, a walk in the park, or whatever – in the middle of it, or when there is a lull in the conversation – reach over and touch her. It can be on the leg, the shoulder, the arm, hand or wherever. Look directly into her eyes and tell her that she is really cute, or that she is really attractive. Wait for her to smile or respond --then ask her if she wants to have sex.

This is so powerful. It's plain, simple and to the point. It lets her know that you are attracted to her, you know what you want and you are not afraid to ask for it. Most likely she wants it too.

Most guys don't have the balls to do this and would never think of doing it in the middle of the first date. Most guys will just beat around the bush and have stupid conversation and wait until the end of the date and try to kiss her or something.

By complimenting her and asking her if she wants to have sex in the middle of the date, it lets her know that you get the whole point of the date. You're not there to just flap your lips and make a new buddy. She's got plenty of these and will probably not waste her time with you anymore, if this is all you do.

It is important to do this in the middle of the date or when the conversation dies. You are a man and she is a woman and there is a reason that you got together. The middle of the date should be the defining moment of it. Timing is very important. If you wait until the end, there is a good chance you will lose your opportunity. Just because she is still with you physically, does not mean that your window of opportunity for sex is still open. Women can close the window very fast, so you have act quickly and at the right time. True, the window, May, open or close several times, but you do not want to take that chance. You want to act as soon as it opens the first time. A, date, is your window of opportunity, and the middle of it, has the biggest opening.

Once again, by touching her, giving her a compliment and asking her if she wants to have sex in the middle of the date, lets her know that you get the whole point that you are together and the whole point of the date. Too many times, guys wait until the end of the date to try to make a move. It shows that they didn't have the guts to do it earlier and the fear of losing their opportunity is now pushing them to do it at the last moment…and she knows this. Women are very intuitive and will pick up on your motivations.

If your date is just coffee or something that can be very quick, then the middle of the date may come sooner than you realize, so, as soon as you get settled, wherever you're at and the conversation dies, initiate this sequence before it's too late.

If she says, yes, then immediately ask her if she is ready to go! Say, "Are you ready to go?" This way, it shows her that you really want her and are excited! If you wait, it doesn't show much enthusiasm and she will probably change her mind, as women so often do. So jump on it while you can!

She may not want to seem too easy and may say, no. If she does, it doesn't necessarily mean that she doesn't want to have sex. She may just be shy or may be shocked that you asked. In this case, ask her to come over for another reason. Ask her to come over for a game of cards or to watch a movie... She may say yes to this. If she does, then most likely she does want to have sex, otherwise, she would not come over after you just asked her for sex. If you want you can wait until the end of the date to ask her to come over for something else. This way, it gives her a chance to think about what you just asked her and wonder if it's going to happen. It may make her want you more and be afraid that you won't ask her again and she may be more receptive by the end of the date... Either way, play with it and see what works best for you.

Interrupt Her
(before she shuts you out)

As I've said before women like to play games and put up resistance. They are not going to just give it to you without a test. One test that I have noticed is when you are with her and talking to her and she is talking excessively, dominating the conversation, or maybe she's acting busy, playing with her phone or doing something. Sometimes, she will keep doing this for a while and then try to end your interaction or date without giving you a chance to say anything.

She could be talking about random things herself or she could be intensely grilling you and asking you a bunch of questions, as in an interview, trying to find out if you stack up to her standards... Whatever the case may be, if you notice this going on and she is talking at a pretty busy pace and dominating the whole conversation...and you just let her, then sometimes, she will come to a stopping point and try to end the date or interaction and say that she has to get going. If you just sit back and let her do this without getting to the point and she ends the interaction and says that she has to go, then she is probably trying to shut you out and testing to see if you really want her bad enough and have the drive and courage to interrupt her and ask for what you want.

Don't wait until the end of the date to stop her and ask for what you want...if you wait until the end, it may be too late. Once she stops and says she has to get going, then it's usually too late. Stop her about midway and go for it.

As the say, it's darkest when you get closer to the light. So, if she is close to giving it up to you, then the more resistance she will probably use and the quicker the window of opportunity will be.

If you are on a date or interacting with a woman and she is doing this, then about midway through the interaction, interrupt her and execute the sequence from the previous section. She is most likely just waiting for you to interrupt and ask for what you want...

If you let her finish and don't stop her, then she will probably shut you out and that may be the last opportunity you will get with her. If she does and you give it another shot after and she doesn't seem interested, you will know why.

What I recommend in this situation is to give it one more try and if she is not budging and completely shutting you out and making excuses why she can't see you, that she is too busy right now, or just not responding when you contact her, then I would completely let it go for a while and maybe hit her up again in a few weeks to a couple months. Sometimes this resets things and she will give you another chance. But if you keep trying to pursue her right after she has shut you out, then you will seem too desperate and she may just block you out for good.

If you wait a while, then hit her up again, she may have been thinking about you, missed you and wondering if she made a mistake. So, in that case, let it go for a while and move on to other women in the meantime.

Initiative
(it's up to you)

It is always best if you can catch signs from her and respond to them because this means that she is already in the mood and wants it. Unfortunately, sometimes you may miss some of the signs or maybe she is a little bit reserved, in which case you may have to take more initiative. If you reach a lull in the conversation and it doesn't seem like things are going much further and you didn't notice any signs, then go ahead and ask her if she wants to come over.

If she doesn't want to, then go ahead and wrap up the date and ask her if she is ready to go. Then walk her to her car and tell her that it was good seeing her and give her a hug and go for a kiss. If she lets you kiss her, then make out with her if you can. If she's cool with this, then there is a good chance she will be open to sex. Ask her if she wants to have sex. If she says no, then say good-bye and let her go.

As soon as you get to your car or within 5 minutes, send her an immediate follow-up text and see if she sends you anything flirty back. If so, follow up right then and give it another shot or hit her up later that night for a booty text. If she doesn't send anything positive or flirty back, then follow up in 2 or 3 days. If you have been communicating through text with her, then use text when you follow up, if voice, then use voice or you can use a combination of the two. Play with it, get a feel for it and see what works best for you.

Physical Contact
(there's nothing more powerful than touch)

Physical contact is one of the most powerful things there is when it comes to turning a woman on. A study was done where there were 2 groups of men at a dance: one group of men approached women and asked them to dance without touching them, the other group went up to women and touched them before asking them to dance. The group who touched the women before they asked them to dance had a 50% higher success rate.

This shows you how powerful touch is. The more physical contact that you make with a woman, while interacting with her, the more likely she will get turned on and want to sleep with you. As I said earlier in this book, I used to do massage therapy and I would say that, maybe, 70 or 80% of the women I massaged would get turned on enough to hit on me.

A perfectly normal form of contact when meeting someone is of course the handshake. Always use this to your advantage. Always shake her hand when you introduce yourself to her. I prefer a nice soft handshake so I can really feel her softness and her feminine energy. To me, it is that sexy feminine energy that turns me on. You can really feel it with some women, especially through the hands. The hands are a very sexy part of the body. It works out perfectly because that is the area that is the most appropriate to touch.

The arms can be great too. As you are shaking her hand, you can also take your other hand and give her arm a slight squeeze. Get into the way that her body feels. Feel her softness and her energy. I also love the feeling of moist skin. I really focus on the feeling of her body. As I focus on that, I feel her feminine energy and it gives me an incredible rush like nothing else. If you can feel this, then she can feel it too and it will turn her on.

Whatever you can feel, she can feel. Take advantage of this and try to get the most succulent feeling that you can when you touch her. This will also tell her that you are a good lover because you have a good touch. Practice every chance you get. This is why I prefer sitting at a bar when I go out with a woman or somewhere where I can be right next to her. This way, I can reach over and touch her as I talk to her.

Massage is also an excellent thing to practice and learn about. Women love massages and massages are the perfect prelude to sex. They really get women turned on and ready to go. You can go straight from doing a massage to having sex with her because you have her at your place and she is already turned on.

Hugs are also an excellent way to get physical contact with her. A lot of times now, when I approach a woman, at the end of our interaction, I will ask her for a hug and a lot of times she will be ok with it. I use this to my advantage and try to really feel the softness of her whole body. Sometimes, she will give me this really big smile afterwards. If this is the case, then go ahead and lean in for a kiss. Why not, if you just made some good physical contact with her and she is turned on and smiling at you, then go for it. If she kisses you back and you start making out with her, then there is a really good possibility that she will come home with you.

Be creative and play with all the different ways you can figure out to get physical contact with women. Explore and see how turned on you can get her right then and there and how far you can take it. Ultimately, that's all it is, just experimenting and going for it and seeing what you can get her to do... The more you do this, the better you will get. It's an art-form and you become an artist by exploring, playing with it and having fun, just like a child!

Being Creative
(part of catching a woman, is using your mind)

Feel free to be creative with your dates. You don't always have to do the same old traditional stuff. You can do anything you want to do and she will appreciate your creativity. It is what will set you apart from other men. The more creative you are, the more it will show her that you are probably an interesting lover too. Just the mention of something different will set you apart, even if she just wants to meet up for coffee or something ordinary, it will stand out to her. Standing out is the key. She could have any ordinary average Joe, but she wants something different, something that she's never had before. Let her know, that you are different.

The whole idea is just to get together, face to face, so you can talk, touch and escalate things to the next level, Sex. So, really, any venue or setting will do. You don't need to meet at some establishment, you can meet her in a park, at the beach, at a pool, or wherever you want. This way too, if she is ok with it, it gives you some privacy and you may feel more at ease going for it.

Sometimes, I feel a little uneasy at a typical small coffee shop because it can sometimes feel like everyone in there can hear you and listen to your conversation. I don't like this. I have certain places that I prefer going because they are a little larger and have more privacy. If the weather is good enough, I like to sit outside. If inside, a large restaurant with booths is probably better than a tiny little coffee shop… Like I said too, a bar or restaurant/bar can be good because of the bar seating where you can sit right next to her. Also, bars tend to be a little dimmer, so it is more relaxing.

A walk is always a good thing because it gives you the ability to talk with her and be side by side and you can always hold hands or stop and kiss and hug. What I like about walks too, is that you have privacy because you are not sitting by a bunch of other people who can hear you. You can meet in nice settings, like a park or by the water or somewhere nice where you can be alone with her out in nature, which in my opinion, is always sexy because it is pure, free and relaxing. It can be inspiring and a turn-on. She may feel more spiritual with you if you are both together in nature. It may inspire her to be more sexual with you and you will have the privacy you need.

As I said earlier too, massage can be excellent foreplay, so take a massage class and then tell her that you need to practice your massage or tell her that you do awesome massages and that you want to give her one. You can also use it on your date if you are somewhere in public, you can ask to see her hand and then give her a hand & arm massage or a shoulder massage…

You can also ask her if she wants to come over and watch a movie or play some cards or any activity that you can think of that would be fun and get her back to your place. That way you are ready to go when something happens!

Be creative and see what you can think of, that is the whole key. Always keep the end in mind and think about where you want things to go and what has to happen next, for that to happen and you will be well on your way. Try to make it as fun and exciting as possible for her, that way she will be intrigued by you and want to follow your suggestions.

Seal the Deal
(Have Sex)

This is what it all comes down to, the whole point, the meaning of this book and our main goal, Sex. Sex is the main thing that we think about when we see a hot woman. It is the main thing that motivates us to pursue a beautiful woman. It is what all of us men fantasize about all day long and want all the time.

Also, the reason sex is so important, is because if you want a woman to be yours, then having sex with her is what's going to seal the deal. It's what is going to grab her emotionally and make her feel attached to you. Everyone wants sex, and if she likes you and is attracted to you, then she is going to want to have sex with you. If she is not necessarily attracted to you, but you give her good sex, then she will become attracted to you and want it again.

If you give her good sex a few times in a row, then she will really get attached to you. This is why sex is so important. Not only does it fulfill a longing, a need that we all have all the time and make us happy and exhilarated, but it connects two people emotionally. Women are especially emotional and sex is very powerful for them. It really gets them into their emotions and their heart, and as they say, "It messes with their head."

If you want a particular woman for a relationship, then it is definitely beneficial to sleep with her as soon as possible, before your chance is gone. If she likes you and wants sex from you and you do not go for it, then she will most likely brush you off anyway. You may as well take your chances while you have them, otherwise, they may be gone for good.

If you don't want to rush it, then just play mister nice guy and go out with her and don't push for sex, but watch for her cues, signaling that she wants it. If she gives you cues that she wants sex, then you should go for it, otherwise, as I said, it may be your last chance.

It's like this, if you want something and you go to a store looking for it and that store doesn't have what you want, then what do you do? You go somewhere else and find it, right? Well, the same thing with a woman. If she wants sex and you don't give it to her, then she is going to go somewhere else and get it. If you like her, then you don't want this to happen because she may get into a relationship with someone else and, bye-bye, there she goes.

The most likely time that sex will occur, is soon after you first meet her. Why is this? Well, this is the most exciting time, when you first meet someone, right? You first see them and you are telling yourself how hot they are and imagining all kinds of naughty things that you would like to do to them, right? Everything is still fresh. There is no emotional baggage built up, nobody has pissed anyone off yet... For all you know, she might be the perfect one, your dream girl, right? This is the perfect time to take advantage of that state, not only in your mind, but also in hers. Plus, after a while, if you don't go for sex, then you run the risk of falling into the buddy-buddy category of hers and you don't want this to happen, otherwise, she will now think of you as a friend and nothing else and it will become that much harder to get inside her, both physically and emotionally.

You can get her either way, but the intent of this book is to go for sex 1st. That way, even if it never turns into a relationship, then at least you had some fun and maybe even made a new fuck friend. That's what happens a lot of times if you give a woman good sex, even if a relationship doesn't happen, you can still see her sexually if she knows that you can satisfy her desires.

Depending on the reason she is coming over to your place, is where you will most likely begin. If you've already asked her to have sex, fun or to just come over and she said yes, without any questions, then you can just go for it straight away when you get back to your place with her. In fact, this is what you should do if sex has already been established; otherwise, she may withdraw her offer to you. Woman are very quick like that, so know what you want and go for it immediately when she gives you the green light.

If you got her to come over because you discussed doing something else first, like playing cards, watching a movie, or giving her a massage, then you will most likely want to start off with that activity and lead into sex from there. Also, it depends on how flirty and playful the conversation was. If it was very flirty, then you could probably go straight into having sex... As stated earlier, voice tone is roughly 35% of communication and body language, 55%.

When you get inside your place, while you are both still standing up, give her a hug then go for a kiss. If she makes out with you, no matter what you had previously discussed doing, then just go for it. If she is enjoying hugging you, then start gently feeling her ass and sniffing around her neck. Tell her that she smells wonderful and just keep inhaling her aroma. For some reason, this really turns women on.

If she is ok with making out and holding each other, then do that for a while and when the moment feels right, start undressing her...reach your hand under her shirt and up her back and undo her bra and start lifting her shirt off and caressing her breasts. The breasts are a huge erogenous zone. Caress her breasts and start sucking on them. Get her nipples really hard and start playing with them. Continue to make out with her here and there. Start feeling the rest of her body, including her ass. Then take off the rest of her clothes. As you remove a piece of her clothing, start taking yours off too. If you take off her shirt, then take yours off too, so everything is pretty equal. That way she doesn't feel awkward that she is the only one exposed.

After you get her clothes mostly or all off, take her over to the bed and lay her down and continue to make out with her and sucking on her breasts. Then take one of your hands and start playing with her pussy and fingering it and playing with her clitoris. If you feel so inclined and you trust that she doesn't have any diseases, then go ahead and eat her out and lick her pussy...focusing mostly on her clitoris. This is the key spot to getting her to have an orgasm, which is the key to giving her great sex and her wanting to see you again...

I'll let you imagine or make up the rest...follow your instincts. If you want to learn more about the actual act of sex or giving great sex, then you may want to do some further research in this area or watch some videos... Porn is always a great and easy way to learn how to give good sex.

You probably should play it safe and use protection so you don't get her pregnant or get any diseases. Do what you feel comfortable with and Have Fun !!! :)

OTHER THINGS

Energy
(it's all connected, use that connection)

Energy is an interesting thing. It is said that all things or everything is energy. I definitely believe this. Energy moves through all things and we are all channels for energy. When you get an idea, thought or inspiration, I believe this to be given to us through energy. Many times, I have been thinking about someone and they have called me or I have run into them. Many times, I have had inspirations to call someone or do something that has worked out perfectly. It's as if this idea to contact them was sent to me and I expressed it and it moved through me to this person and got the desired result. Never underestimate the power that lies behind an idea, inspiration or thought that you may have. It may be just the right time to carry it out, and when we follow it, that force works for us.

Another interesting thing or technique that I use sometimes, is, I focus on my heart and feel the energy or pulsation around that area. Generally, when I feel an intense feeling in this area and it is pulsing heavily, I know that there is someone out there, usually a woman that I am interested in, that is thinking about me and feeling the same sensation. Usually, it is the woman that I happen to be thinking about right then that I can't take my mind off of. This has confirmed itself many times with women that I was dating at the moment and as I felt this sensation grow in strength, they then contacted me. I believe women, in general, are much more in-tune with this than men. If you focus enough, you too, can learn to harness this ability.

If you then focus on it and let that intense feeling grow, you can attract women to you through this energy. The more they are, "feeling you," naturally, the more responsive they will be towards you, as women very much follow their hearts!

When you are interested in a woman, think about her as intensely as you can and focus on the energy around your heart and continue to focus on it and notice the intensity of that feeling grow. Hang on to that feeling as long as you can and watch what happens.

You may particularly want to try this after you have contacted her and left a message, text, email…and are waiting for a reply from her, or even if you called and hung up. As long as she knows it was from you. Focus on that intense feeling around your heart and as it grows and gets more intense, the more you will be connected with her and she will literally feel you. The more this feeling grows, the more likely that she will feel compelled to contact you.

Everything is energy and whatever you focus on, you will pull towards you with that energy. The more intensely you feel it in your heart, the stronger it will pull. So, focus, focus, focus and feel.

Tension = Attraction
(coming together is more likely, if there is intrigue)

In order to attract something to you, there has to be tension. Tension is what pulls things towards us. It's like wrapping a rubber band around something and having the other end in your hand. The more tension that is in the rubber band, the more it will pull that object towards us.

Tension is that intense feeling of energy around the heart area as described in the Energy section. The stronger and more intense those heart feelings get, the stronger the tension or pulling power to attract whatever it is that we are thinking about, including women.

Another technique and way to describe, "Attraction," would be the teeter-totter model or tit for tat. Some people feel that when you take an action towards a female, that you wait for her to reciprocate and take the next action, so everything remains balanced. So, if two people are on a teeter-totter and are balanced, then if one moves forward towards the other person, there then becomes tension or pressure for the other person to reciprocate for balance to remain. Once the other person reciprocates, then you take another step closer to them and wait for them to reciprocate. The farther you get into this process the more tension there will be for each other to reciprocate and continue until you both come together. No pun intended. ;)

While you are waiting for the other person to reciprocate, focus on that energy around the heart area and continue to focus on it until it grows and becomes more and more intense and pulsates stronger and stronger. As you do this, keep the woman that you are waiting to make the next move, in mind. If the energy pulsations around your heart get really intense then you will know that she is feeling it too. As you continue to focus on this, it will keep those feelings in her as well and she will feel much more compelled to respond.

In general, I tend to focus on my heart energy even though I may not have a specific woman in mind, or even when my mind is flipping back and forth and thinking about multiple women. I will continue to focus on that energy and as it remains strong, I feel it is much more likely to connect with a woman's energy and pull her towards me even though I don't know which one it will be. Sometimes, as I do this, the pulsations will get very strong and I will know my vibes have caught someone else's and are pulling them towards me. It's like a fishing line that has caught something and you cannot see beneath the water what it is yet, but it is pulling them closer and closer to you because you can feel it. Then, sometimes, the woman that it has caught will surface and contact me.

In-Person
(being together is the whole point)

I feel that your chances of succeeding with a woman in person are far greater than trying to score online or indirectly, at least initially when you first meet her. There is nothing like when you are face to face and she doesn't have much choice but to respond to you. On the phone or online…she can always ignore you and not respond. In person, she is more obligated to respond, so you have more of a chance.

Also, in person, you get a lot of clues that you don't get online or over the phone. You can see her body language, facial expressions and tone of voice and you can feel her vibes if you are sensitive enough. Even if you don't succeed right then, you can get clues from all these things that she is expressing both consciously and unconsciously and learn from them if you pay attention.

You can also approach as many women as you want. You can go to shopping malls, walk through all the stores and departments, colleges, gyms, downtown, flea markets, events, anywhere there is women, you can go and approach them. You can do as little or as much as you like, as long as there are women to hit on.

The best part to me is that I don't have to go out of my way to meet women. I simply go about my normal, everyday business and when I see a hot lady that I want to have sex with, I approach her and talk to her.

The other great thing is that when you approach women in your local city or area, most likely, they live close by. If you meet someone online, who knows where they live, it can be really far away. Personally, I will not drive more than 1 hour to see someone and preferably no more than 30 minutes. If it's farther than that, it's too far and a waste of my time and resources and too inconvenient.

The Moment
(it all happens right now)

It all boils down to this one moment that we are always eternally in right now! Sex and everything else always happens right now, not sometime in the future or past, the only thing that is real is right now. Women are really creatures of the moment. They want you to catch them right now in this moment when they are ready for it and feeling it.

If they are feeling it right now and you do not act on it, then they do not want to commit to giving it to you in the future. If you cannot satisfy them now, then they will think, *how is he going to satisfy me in the future or why would he satisfy me in the future?* If you cannot demonstrate to her that you have the ability to recognize that she is turned on and wants it now, then how will you catch it in the future?

I know that this is not always true, because people do learn and grow, but women do not always think like that. If you miss an opportunity now, then she may not give you another opportunity. If she does, she may make it twice as challenging for you the next time. This is why you want to be as sharp and alert as you can, at each moment, and catch her right off the bat. Plus, when you first meet a woman, this is the most probable time that fast sex will occur because of the initial excitement of her meeting someone new and being curious about them, before any negative or unpleasant associations have occurred. So you always want to go for it right away…in this moment.

If a woman is in a relationship, then she may only give you, this moment. She may not feel good about making any plans with another guy since she is already in a relationship. This is another reason that she may not give you her number or contact information either... However, if it just happens in the moment, then she can justify it to herself by thinking that she did not plan it, that it just, "Happened."

Women think like this. They are very good at compartmentalizing things and keeping them separate in their mind. So, if it falls into the spur-of-moment-just-happened-without-thinking-fun-but-I-will-not-do-it-again category, then it may be ok. Or they may even justify it in their mind more-so by telling themselves that they were broken up with their boyfriend at the time...or that they just had, "Coffee," with you...

Another interesting thing about the way that life is designed is that it is always pushing us to grow, by challenging us. If we step up to the challenges, then life will reward us and give us something new. If we don't, then we create our own punishment by having to go through the drudgery of the, "Same ol', same ol'." Happiness or satisfaction sustains itself when we are constantly progressing. Reaching our goals is always nice and a good feeling, but it won't last. We have to keep moving and progressing.

Always take a look around you and see how you can progress at this moment. What challenges is life offering you right now? A lot of times, if you want to get laid, life will offer you a challenge to catch something that you have never caught before or push through a boundary that you never been through, first. Sometimes, it is that last step that we didn't take, that will lead us to getting what we want, including sex. Open your eyes and trust your instincts and look for the opportunity at this moment to push past your boundaries and do something that you have never done before. Ask yourself, am I doing all that I can here or is there something else that I can do? Sometimes, as you are walking away from a woman, you will get an insight, a flash of what you should have done. Don't be afraid to turn around and go back and give it another try. If you walk away and pass that opportunity by, then that may be the last time she gives you that opportunity. Life has a funny way of working this way, so you have to constantly push your boundaries at every moment to get the results that you want. So, if you feel that you can't go any further, then push a little bit more. This is when you get the most growth.

Break Apart
(make her want you)

Sometimes, when you make your first initial contact with a woman and are going for it and she is not giving you the response that you want, it can sometimes be powerful to create a little separation.

Say, you are both somewhere where you'll be lingering around for a little while, like the store, the gym, a festival or wherever…you can walk away and continue to do what you were doing before you met her and see if she remains in close proximity to you. If you notice her lingering around after you just hit on her, then there is a good chance that she may want you to continue to pursue her, or to chase after her…

By giving her some space and not being afraid to separate from her, shows her that you are secure with yourself and are not attached to the outcome. Sometimes, when she sees this, she will become more attracted to you and want you.

Also, it gives her a chance to think about what just happened. Maybe it happened too fast and she just responded defensively automatically. Now, being separated for a few minutes, she may have time to think about where you were going with it and it may turn her on the more she thinks about it…

So give her a few minutes and if you notice her still around and maybe even glancing at you, then definitely approach her and go for it again... Sometimes it happens on the second or third try. Women like to play this game sometimes to see if you want her enough and have the confidence to persist. As they say, 3 is the magic number.

Letting it Go
(move on)

For our purposes here, it's all about getting sex fast. We are not here to take weeks or months to get sex from someone. We are here to catch the fruit when it is ripe and eat it. It's all a numbers game. It's that 1 or 2, maybe 3 out of 10 that want it. It's catching them when they are ready for it and seizing the opportunity. We are not trying to date someone or court them or waste a lot of time to get sex. Our goal is to simply catch them when they are ready and enjoy the opportunity while it lasts.

Sometimes, we may come across someone who appeared that they might be ready to have some fast sex, but it turned out they were not, or maybe we didn't make the exact right move at the exact right time and then they became more resistant and the opportunity became more of a hassle than it was worth... In these instances, we have to know when to draw the line and let it go.

If it's starting to seem like more work than it is enjoyment, then it's probably time to let it go. Our technique is not about putting a lot of effort forward and spending a lot of time trying to get it. We are simply looking for the ones that are ready to give it up right now and jumping on the opportunity. So, if you are no longer enjoying the process with someone, then just let it go and move on to the next piece of fruit that looks ripe.

You Never Know
(when you least expect it)

Life has a funny way of giving us something when we finally give up or are not trying anymore. If you are getting tired of trying, then just let it go for a while and see what might pop up when you least expect it. If you do see an opportunity right in front of your face, when you are not even looking for it, then go for it.

This happens to me all the time. I have learned that it's not worth the hassle to have the constant pressure on myself of always looking for it and trying everywhere I go, but a funny thing happens when I don't care anymore and am not looking for it. It appears right there in front of me and I instantly get heated up and go for it automatically.

After a while, you approach so many women that it will just become automatic to you. You will instantly see a hot woman and, Boom, you just have to go for it! Something kicks in, like a turbo-boost or something…it's weird…and you feel like you have to go for it. So you do, and you never know, it may happen when you are least expecting it!

PUTTING IT ALL TOGETHER (10 Scenarios)

These are scenarios showing what is possible using this method and how it all works:

Scenario 1

You are at the grocery store shopping for food. You are in the produce section getting your vegetables and fruits. You hit on a couple different women but they are cold and brush you off. You continue shopping. Now you are in one of the food aisles and are looking at different items on the shelves. You notice a lady that you didn't talk to in the produce section and she is now in the same aisle as you and looking at items nearby. You take this as a possible sign that she is trying to get your attention by being in close proximity to you. She's pretty attractive so you decide to approach her. The interaction goes as follows:

You: "Hi, my name's _____. I thought you looked really cute and wanted to say, hi."

She seems friendly and says,

Her: "Oh, Hi!"

You: "What's your name?"

Her: "I'm Cathy"

You put out your hand and shake hers.

You: "Nice to meet you!"

You: "I was just wondering if you would join me for some coffee?"

She smiles and says,

"I'm kind of busy today. I can't. But thanks for asking!"

You: "Can I get your number?"

She smiles and says, "Next time!"

Since she smiled and said the keyword, "Next time," you say,

"Wanna come over?"

Her: "What do you have in mind?"

You smile and say, "Wanna have some fun?"

Her: "Where do you live?"

You: "Just down the street. You wanna come?"

Her: "Ok!"

You: "Are you ready to go?"

Her: "Yah, sure. Do you need to finish shopping?"

You: "No, that's ok. Let's go."

Her: "Ok."

You both walk outside and you tell her to follow you to your house and get her phone number in case she gets lost from you. She follows you to your house and you have amazing sex!

Scenario 2

You are at the gym around midnight. You just finished your workout and took a shower and are on your way out. In the last row of cardio machines, you see a hot young girl by herself working out. You decide to approach her. You go up to her and tap her on the shoulder. She takes off her headphones and looks at you.

You: "Hi, my name is _____. I just thought you looked really cute and wanted to come and say, hi."

She smiles and says, "Hi."

You: "Do you work out here often?"

Her: "Once or twice a week."

You: "What's your name?"

Her: "I'm Melanie"

You put out your hand, smile and shake her hand.

You: "I was just wondering if you would join me for a drink?"

Her: "I just got here"

You: "Can I get your number?"

Her: "I have a boyfriend"

You: "Do you wanna be friends?"

She gets big smile on her face and says, "That's inappropriate."

Since she gave you a big flirty smile when she said that, you smile and say,

"You wanna come over?"

Her: "Where?"

You: "My place."

Her: "For?"

You: "Do you like massages?"

Her: "No, I'm ticklish."

You smile and say, "You wanna have some fun?"

She smiles and says, "Ok"

You: "Are you ready to go?"

Her: "Yah"

You both walk outside and she follows you to your house and you bang.

Scenario 3

You are in a clothing store just browsing around. You are walking through different aisles and seeing what they have. You approach 3 different women, but no luck. Then you spot this really hot young lady who is looking at some items. You walk over to her and say,

"Hi, my name's_____. I just thought you looked really cute and wanted to come say, hi."

Her: "Hi"

You: "What's your name?"

Her: "I'm Elaine"

You put out your hand and shake hers.

You: "I'm _____, nice to meet you!"

She smiles and you ask her what she is shopping for and get into a little conversation for a few minutes. You find out that she has just moved to town and is shopping to decorate her new place. The conversation dies down and you say,

"I was wondering if you would join me for some coffee?"

Her: "I can't, I have to decorate my place today."

You: "Can I get your number?"

Her: "Why don't you give me yours."

You: "If I call your phone, then you'll have my number in your phone."

She smiles and says, ok. She gives you her number and you call her phone... You tell her to have a good day and to have fun decorating her place. She gives you an especially flirty smile and wave and says thanks! You walk out of the store. As soon as you get outside, you send her the following text message:

"Great meeting you, Elaine! Have a good day! :) (your name)"

She texts back, "You too!!! :)"

Noticing her flirtatious body language when you said good bye and her overwhelming enthusiasm in her text response with the exclamation points and smiley face, you text the following,

"Wanna come over? :)"

Her: "I have to finish decorating."

You: "Wanna have some fun? ;)"

Her: "Ok"

You: "Are you ready to go?"

Her: "Sure"

You: "K. meet me in front of the store"

Her: "K. be there in a minute"

She meets you outside, follows you to your place and you fuck!

Scenario 4

It is Saturday afternoon around 3 pm and you are at the gym. You just finished working out and are relaxing in the sauna. This hot petite lady walks in and sits across from you and lies down. You move over next to her and start a conversation just asking general questions about her. You find out that she was a massage therapist.

You say, "I'm really good at giving massages. You wanna come over for a massage?"

Her: "I have to go somewhere after this."

You: "Can I get your number?"

Her: "I can't."

You: "What do you have planned this afternoon?"

Her: "I give dance lessons down the street."

You: "Oh, that sounds cool. Well, it was good meeting you!"

You get up to leave and she sits up, gives you this big flirty smile, sticks out her hand to shake yours and says, "What was your name?"

You tell her your name and she says, "See you soon!"

Since she shows a lot of interest by sitting up, smiling, shaking your hand and saying the key phrase, "See you soon," you say,

"You wanna come over?"

She smiles and says, "Ok!"

You: "Are you ready to go?"

Her: "Sure."

You: "I'll meet you out front in 15 minutes, Ok?"

Her: "Ok"

You both leave the sauna, go shower and meet her up front. She follows you to your place and you bang.

Scenario 5

You are going to the gym to workout and you just pulled into the parking lot and parked. It is Thursday afternoon around 2 pm. You get out of your car and start walking across the parking lot towards the front door. At the same time, you see this hot lady walking past you to her car. She had sunglasses on, but you felt this really strong vibe as she past by and you couldn't help but turn your head and look at her. Something is pulling you towards her, so you go with it and follow her and catch her as she is opening her car door and say,

"Hi, my name is _____. You look really cute, I just had to come and say, hi."

She gives a big smile and says, hi.

You: "What's your name?"

Her: "I'm Monique"

You smile and say, "Nice meeting you, Monique!"

You put out your hand and shake her hand and say,

"I was wondering if you want to grab some coffee with me?"

Her: "I can't. I'm supposed to meet my friends right now."

You: "Can I get your number?"

Her: "I'm in a relationship."

You: "You wanna be friends?"

She gives you a big smile and says, Ok.

You say, "What's the best way to contact you?"

Her: "I guess I can give you my number."

You whip out your phone and call her number so she has your number in her phone. You smile and tell her that it was good meeting her and say good-bye. She gives you a big smile and says, "Bye!" You start walking towards the gym. As you are walking away from her, you feel this incredible pull towards her. It's hard to walk away and you want to text her immediately. You walk just out of view and send the following text message:

"It was good meeting you, Monique! Have a good day! :) (your name)"

She texts you right back, "Good meeting you too. I'm usually pretty busy, so I'll probably just see you around the gym."

Some women don't like to give many clues in their texts and keep them pretty dry. They want you to figure it out for yourself, be confident and know what you want... She is giving you resistance right off the bat, but if you read into it and notice how she said she will probably just "see you around..." That is one of our keywords which means she might be available now, but be testing you and trying to fool you out of it. The fact that she text-messaged you back immediately is a HUGE sign! In most cases, this probably means that she is available right now... Also, combined with the incredibly strong vibe that you were feeling when you first saw her and when you walked away from her... All of this, tells you to hit her back immediately. So, you text the following:

"Wanna come over? :)"

Her: "Where do you live?"

You: "About 10 minutes away. Follow me, ok?

Her: "Ok"

You walk back over to her car and tell her where you are parked and that you will pull your car around so she can follow you. You both go back to your place and fuck.

Scenario 6

You are at the mall walking around on a Friday around 3 pm looking to meet someone. You hit on a few women but no luck. You walk into the big book store, use the bathroom and look around a little bit. You approach a couple more women, but again, no luck. Then you notice that they have a coffee shop in the bookstore and you spot this really hot looking young college girl with her laptop computer. She is dressed kind of fancy but also sexy, with a short skirt and a business type suit on. You walk over to her and tap her on the shoulder. She looks up at you and takes her headphones off and you say,

"Hi, I thought you looked really cute and wanted to come say, hi."

She smiles and says, "Hi"

You: "I was wondering if I could join you?"

Her: "Sure" and she clears some space for you to sit next to her.

You sit down and start a little conversation and ask if she is doing schoolwork… She says, yes. You ask her where she goes to school and what subjects she is studying and what she wants to do when she graduates… She elaborates. You find a few commonalities with what she is saying and tell her about them. You ask her where she lives. She tells you she lives at the local college. She says that she has a lot of, "Stress."

Her: "Where do you live?"

You: "Oh, just down the street. You wanna come over?"

Her: "I've got to get this done, but I'm sure I'll see you soon!" She smiles.

You: "Can I get your number?"

Her: "Sure, it's …"

You whip out your cell phone and enter her number. You smile, tell her it was good meeting her and that you'll talk to her soon. You walk out of the bookstore and send her the following text message:

"It was good meeting you! Have a good day! (your name) :)"

She texts back, "it was good meeting you too. have a good day"

Since she didn't put any exclamation points, return a smiley face, or anything that gives an overwhelming sign that she wants to hook up right now and since you already asked if she wanted to come over and she declined, but said she's sure that she'll see you soon, you decide to wait until later that night and send her a booty text.

(You could have tried to push through her resistance in the coffee shop after you asked her to come over, when she said that she had to get her work done, but that she's sure that she will "see you soon." And she did mention the keyword, "stress." You could have asked her right then if she wanted to have some fun or sex…but since you didn't, you'll send her a booty text tonight).

At 10:33 pm, you send the following text:

"What are you doing?"

Her: "School work"

You: "Wanna come over?"

Her: "What'd you have in mind???"

You: "Just a little fun ;) U down?"

Her: "Like what???"

You: "Wanna have sex?"

Her: "I don't think so"

She may be giving some extra resistance here because you didn't ask her earlier in the coffee shop when she may have already been ready to go… So, she may have stepped up her resistance this time to make it a little more challenging to see if you have the confidence and if you really know what you want now…

You: "How about a game of cards?"

Her: "Ok. Where do you live?"

You text her your address and she comes over. You offer her a glass of wine but she declines. You sit down on your couch and play some Uno. Just a simple game that she can pick up on easily…nothing too complicated. Just something that gives you a little back and forth action that you can tease each other and build some sexual tension with…

Obviously, since you asked her to have sex, even though she said no, yet she still came over after knowing your intentions and based on the overall interactions with her and how fast everything happened, she probably really does want sex, but is just playing a little hard to get. After about 10 or 15 minutes of playing and teasing, you lean over and give her a kiss and start making out with her. Things quickly escalate. You take her clothes off and have sex.

Scenario 7

It's about 10 pm on a Sunday night. You walk into the gym to go workout. You are walking to the men's locker room to put your bag in the locker. On your way there, you walk behind a row of cardio equipment. You spot this hot girl on a stairmaster. She has the finest ass you have ever seen! You just have to approach her! You go up behind her and tap her on the arm. She steps down off the stairmaster and you say,

"I just thought you looked really cute and had to come and say, hi."

She smiles and says, "Hi"

You: "I was wondering if you would join me for a drink?"

Her: "Not tonight"

You: "What's your name?"

Her: "Amy"

You: "Hi, I'm _____."

You put your hand out and shake her hand softly, feeling her sensuality. She gives you a really big flirty smile!

You: "Can I get your number?"

Her: "Ok"

You get your cell phone out and say, "Ok. What's your number?"

You put her number in your cell phone and call hers so that she now has your number too. You smile and tell her that it was good meeting her and that you will talk to her later. She smiles and says good-bye. After you get to the locker room, it slips your mind to send an immediate follow-up text and you change and go work out.

The next day, Monday, around 2 pm you give her a voice call and leave her the following message in friendly tone, "Hi Amy, it's _____, from the gym last night, just calling to see if you want to get together for some coffee. Give me a call. Hope you're having a good day! Bye!"

She calls you back in about an hour and you answer the phone, "Hey, how are you?"

Her: "Hey, sorry I missed your call. I just got out of class."

You: "That's cool. Hey, I was just wondering if you wanna get together for some coffee?"

Her: "Sure. I can meet you at the coffee shop by the gym at 4pm."

You: "Ok, great! I'll see you then!"

Her: "Ok. See you then!"

You pull up to the coffee shop at 4 pm and see her walking in. You catch up to her, say hi and get in line to order your coffee. She asks you where you live and you ask her if she wants to come over. She smiles, but shakes her head and says lets get some coffee. You ask her what she wants and order for the both of you. You pay for the coffee and find a quiet table by the window. She starts asking you questions about yourself. She continues talking for a while, so you just listen and acknowledge what she is saying and answer her questions... Then, after a while she quiets down and is smiling, and gripping her coffee cup with both hands and nervously twisting them around it (this is a good sign) and she asks you if you have any questions for her. (Most likely she is nervous because she has opened herself up to the possibility of having sex at this moment and is feeling vulnerable because of it. These moments are fast windows that you have to recognize immediately and take advantage of, or they will be gone quickly! You've put together the pieces: the flirtatious smile at the gym, her asking you where you live, & her nervously gripping her coffee cup while she smiles & asks you if you have any questions for her...). So, with a big smile you say,

"Do you wanna have sex?" She smiles excitedly and says Ok.

You ask her, "Are you ready to go?"

She says yes and you both walk out. You find out that she doesn't have a car, so you both get into your car. You look over at her and she is smiling nervously at you. You lean over and give her a kiss and start making out. She is very excited and wants it badly. You take off and drive to your place. On the way, you hold hands a little bit and kiss now and then at stop lights... You get to your place and immediately come together with her and start making out passionately and taking her clothes off. She is driving you crazy and you are both totally excited and you make passionate love...

Scenario 8

It is a Saturday evening about 7 pm and you have just finished picking up a couple items at the grocery store. You just get in your car and you see this really hot lady walk by with a bag of groceries. She's going to her car. You get out of your car and you walk over to her. She is putting her groceries in her trunk. You walk up and say,

"Hi, my name is _____. I just thought you looked really cute and had to come and say, hi."

She smiles and says hi.

You: "I was wondering if you would join me for some coffee?"

Her: "I've got to get home, we're making crab cakes."

You: "How about tomorrow?"

Her: "I'm dating someone."

You: "Can I get your number?"

She smiles and says ok. You ask what her name is, tell her yours and shake her hand. You whip out your cell phone and put her number in. You tell her to enjoy her crab cakes and walk back to your car and get in. You send her this immediate follow-up text:

"Good meeting you! Have a good weekend! :) (your name)"

She doesn't respond. The next day, Sunday, around noon you call her and leave the following voice message in an upbeat friendly tone:

"Hey Cindy, it's _____ from the supermarket yesterday, just seeing if you wanna grab some coffee with me. Hope you're having a good day! Call me. Bye!"

She sends you the following text message, "Hey, kinda busy today"

You text back, "Ok. ttyl"

You wait until Tuesday evening around 9 pm and text the following message, "Hey, what are you doing?"

She texts back, "Reading."

You: "Wanna come over?"

Her: "I feel like a movie"

You: "Wanna come over and watch a movie?"

Her: "No, what's playing in the theatre?"

You: "I don't know. Let me see…"

You look up online to see what is playing and then you let her know. You both decide on a movie and meet her there. You get into the theatre and sit down. You look over at her and she is smiling at you. You lean over and start making out with her. You watch the movie and make out here and there during it.

Afterwards, you ask if she wants to come over and she says, no. You walk her to her car and start making out with her. She says, "Let's sit in the car for a little bit." You say ok and she parks in a private spot away from other cars. You recline the seats and continue making out and talking. This continues for about an hour and you are getting really turned on. You tell her that you want her. She smiles and shakes her head. Remembering that she said she was dating someone, you say,

"How about just one time?"

She says, "Are you sure?"

You say yes and she agrees to come over. She drops you off at your car and follows you home and you have sex.

Scenario 9

It is a Friday afternoon and you are at the gym and just finished your workout and took a shower. You are walking out of the men's locker room. You see this really hot thin lady laying down, working out on the abs machine, you decide to approach her. You wait until she has stopped and is resting. You walk over and kneel down on the floor next to her and say,

"Hi, I just thought you looked really cute and wanted to come over and say, hi."

Her: "Oh, Hi"

You ask her how often she comes to the gym and start a little conversation with her. Then you ask what her name is and shake her hand. Then you say, "Hey, I was just wondering if you wanna grab a drink with me?" She says that she can't because she has got to prepare for a party she's throwing tomorrow. You ask for her number, she says, "sure," and you put it in your phone. You smile and tell her that you will talk to her soon, then you get up and leave.

When you get to your car, you send the following immediate follow-up text message, "It was good meeting you, Sherry! Have a good day. (your name)" You don't get any response from her. So, you call her on Sunday instead of the next day because she said that she is throwing a party the next day. You call her around noon and she answers.

You: "Hi, how are you?"

Her: "Hi, I'm good."

You: "How was your party yesterday?"

Her: "It was good."

You: "Hey, I was just wondering if you wanna get some coffee with me?"

Her: "Actually, we're still partying. We're going out to dinner tonight."

You: "How about a drink later tonight?"

Her: "I'm kind of busy on the weekends."

You: "When's good for you?"

Her: "I'm not sure."

You: "Ok. Well have a good day! Talk to you later."

Her: "Bye!"

Since she didn't respond to your immediate follow-up text and sounds kind of busy and doesn't want to make any type of commitment, you decide to wait a few days and hit her up later in the week with a late night booty text.

You wait until Thursday evening at 10:33 pm and send the following text message:

"What are you doing?"

Her: "At the gym. Done working out." (10:40 pm)

You: "Wanna come over? :)" (10:44 pm)

Her: "I'm driving now. Can't text. Have to get up early for a meeting tomorrow. Have a good night!" (11:33 pm)

She puts up a little resistance, but she responds this time and fairly quickly and gives you a couple clues. She tells you to have a good night with an exclamation point at the end and responds exactly one hour later at 11:33 (very good signs!).

You: "Wanna have sex? :)" (12:33)

Her: "Where do you live?" (12:34)

You: "(your address)" (12:35)

Her: "Ok :)" (12:36)

Her: "Be there in 30 min" (12:37)

You: "K. See u then :)"   (12:38)

She comes over and you get it on...

Scenario 10

This scenario is a variation on Scenario 5. This time you are fooled by her response to your immediate follow up text-message and because she said she was busy right now and going to meet some friends...so you don't try to push through her resistance (which of course, you should always do, so you don't miss out on opportunities that may not be there later!)

You are going to the gym to workout and you just pulled into the parking lot and parked your car. It is Thursday afternoon around 2 pm. You get out and start walking across the parking lot towards the front door. At the same time, you see this hot lady walking past you to her car. She had sunglasses on, but you felt this really strong vibe as she past by and couldn't help but turn your head and notice her. Something is pulling you towards her, so you go with it and follow her and catch her as she is opening her car door and say,

"Hi, my name is _____. You look really cute, I just had to say, hi."

She gives a big smile and says, hi.

You: "What's your name?"

___

Her: "I'm Monique"

You smile and say, "Nice meeting you!" You put out your hand and shake her hand and say,

"I was wondering if you want to grab some coffee with me?"

Her: "I can't. I supposed to meet my friends right now."

You: "Can I get your number?"

Her: "I'm in a relationship."

You: "You wanna be friends?"

She gives you a big smile and says, Ok.

You say, "What's the best way to contact you?"

Her: "I guess I can give you my number."

You whip out your cell phone and call her number so she has your number in her phone. You smile and tell her that it was good meeting her and say good-bye. She gives you a big smile and says, "Bye!" You start walking towards the gym. As you are walking away from her, you feel this incredible pull towards her. It's hard to walk away and you want to text her immediately. You walk just out of view and send the following text message:

"It was good meeting you, Monique! Have a good day! :) (your name)"

She texts back right away, "Good meeting you too. I'm usually pretty busy, so I'll probably just see you around the gym."

Since she said that she was busy and had to go meet some friends right now and because of her text message saying that she will probably just see you around, you decide to let it go for now and not pursue her any further today (you are ignoring the really intense vibes that you are feeling from her and the fact that she texted you back immediately! Not good, but that is what you decide).

Since you saw her yesterday at the gym around 2 pm, you assume that maybe she is off during the daytime and you text her the next day, Friday, the following message around noon:

"Wanna grab some coffee?"

She responds, "I'm out of town this weekend."

So, you wait until after the weekend to text her again. Tuesday you send the following text message around 11 am:

"How was your weekend?"

She doesn't respond. So, you wait until Thursday and send the following text around noon:

"What are you doing?"

Again, no response.   You decide to give it a break and let it go until next week. The following Tuesday rolls around and you decide that since she is not responding to the text messages, to step it up and call her so she might feel more of a connection to you by hearing your voice again. If she doesn't answer, you will leave a nice flirty voice message. She doesn't answer, so you leave the following voice message in a sexy tone:

"Hi Monique, it's _____. I just wanted to let you know that I'm really good at giving massages and was just wondering if you wanna come over for a massage."

Just after you leave the voice message, you send her this text message, "How are you? :)"

She texts you back in a few minutes, "Hey, I'm a little busy this week. I should have more time next week :)"

You: "Ok. Have a good week!"

The signs are telling you that she is not interested in a relationship, since she already has one and since she did not want to get together for coffee, yet she smiled and said yes to being friends, giving you her number and responding positively after your voice message… The only thing left is sex, and since she seems too busy during the day, you decide to hit her up with a late night booty text 2 days later on Thursday night at 11:33.

You text her: "What are u doing?"

She responds in a few minutes, "Reading"

You: "You want that massage?"

Her: "I don't think I need a massage."

Some resistance to see if she can trick you out of it...

You: "Wanna come over?"

Her: "What are you thinking???"

A little possible intimidation with 3 question marks…

You: "Just a little fun before bed ;) lol"

She doesn't respond, so 10 minutes later you send the following text:

"Wanna have sex? :)"

Her: "Where do you live?"

You: "(your address)"

Her: "Who do you live with?"

You: "No one. I have my own place."

She doesn't respond, so 10 minutes later you send the following:

"You wanna come"

Her: "Ok"

Her: "I'll be there at 1"

You: "Ok"

It's about 1:10 am and you don't see her yet, so you text her:

"You coming?"

Her: "Be there in 5 minutes"

She shows up and you have amazing sex!

Keep in mind that these scenarios and the methods in this book are possibilities. It doesn't mean that these are going to happen every time you meet women. It is a numbers game and you will most likely only get a small percentage of them. Don't hold on to any expectations, just go out there and play with the methods. Experiment with them, revise them & develop your own techniques to add to them as well. These are just some things that I have learned that would have made the whole process much easier and put me much further ahead if I would have known them from the beginning. Ultimately, you will have to experiment and find what works for you. This is what works for me at times. The only way to succeed is to try. You won't have successes if you aren't willing to fail miserably at first. The idea is to have fun with it! Enjoy the process! Women are fun to interact with and it is an exciting challenge to pursue them. If you are enjoying the process, then women will enjoy interacting with you and you will be much more likely to succeed. Women will even give you clues to help you out, so watch for them and keep learning and improving all the time. Satisfaction with anything is not in the end result, but in the constant progress towards it.

If you go out there with the attitude of just enjoying what you are doing and having fun with it, then no matter what the result is, you are a success. If you keep taking notes of what you are doing and reflect back on each situation, taking note of what you did and how she responded and watch for little clues and what you can do better the next time and keep improving, then you will eventually reach your goal. Then, once it starts happening, it will become easier and easier, just like riding a bike! :)

Have fun & enjoy!

If you enjoyed the book, please leave a favorable review wherever you bought it.

Thank You!

If you have any questions, comments, or stories
you'd like to share, feel free to email me.

Sky@GetSexFast.Org